Contents

Diagnosing Cancer
in
Primary Care

Radcliffe Medical Press Ltd
18 Marcham Road, Abingdon, Oxon OX14 1AA

British Library Cataloguing in Publication Data

A catalogue record for this book is available from the British Library.

ISBN 1 85775 307 0

Typeset by Acorn Bookwork, Salisbury, Wiltshire
Printed and bound by Biddles Ltd, Guildford and King's Lynn

Preface

This handbook is a concise, primary-care guide, which outlines epidemiological data, risk factors, symptoms, and signs of the more common cancers, along with the place and value of investigations both for presymptomatic and symptomatic conditions.

It is written from the perspective of a general practitioner who has a particular interest in the rational diagnosis and assessment of patients in a primary-care setting. However, it is important to appreciate that primary care, as the 'first point of contact with the National Health Service' is much broader than general practice. A patient's initial encounter may be with a pharmacist, nurse, health visitor, midwife, a member of the general practice administrative staff, dentist, optician, or even the hospital-based casualty department. Patients with a chronic cough often visit the pharmacist on a number of occasions before making an appointment with the general practitioner. Women frequently discuss breast and gynaecological symptoms with health visitors or practice nurses. It is well known that patients are very loath to consult their general practitioner about rectal bleeding. Consequently, I hope this book is helpful to all my primary-care clinical colleagues.

The Calman–Hine report emphasised three areas of importance for cancer services – the cancer centre, the cancer unit, and primary care. This book focuses on one of the aspects of primary-care oncology that is of great concern to many of us working in primary care – **making the diagnosis of cancer**.

Nicholas Summerton
May 1999

Acknowledgements

I should like to express my thanks to the many friends and colleagues in Huddersfield, Halifax, and Hull who have helped, guided, and supported me in the development of this book.

I am also particularly grateful to the following individuals:

- Heidi Allen from Radcliffe Medical Press for encouraging me to write the book
- Sara Mann for typing the manuscript and for coping patiently with endless amendments
- Emily Summerton for checking my sums in Chapter 2
- Keith Hopcroft for his very helpful review of the original manuscript
- Linda Bell, Scunthorpe Trust Librarian, for her efficiency, help, and patience, answering my requests for large numbers of references
- Alan Brook, Karen Dean, Bert Jindall, and John Hicks for helping me to develop some of the ideas contained in this book
- Keith Finney, Sheila Finney, John Clayden, John Priestman, John Standring, and Bob Higson: my trainers from Holmfirth and Kirkburton who first opened my eyes to the real nature of clinical general practice.

Above all I should like to acknowledge the support of my family – Ailie, Emily, Siân, and Katrina.

List of abbreviations

AFP	α-fetoprotein
ALL	acute lymphoblastic leukaemia
ALT	alanine aminotransferase
AML	acute myeloid leukaemia
BCC	basal-cell carcinoma
BPH	benign prostatic hyperplasia
CA-125	cancer antigen 125
CEA	carcinoembryonic antigen
CIN	cervical intraepithelial neoplasia
CLL	chronic lymphocytic leukaemia
CML	chronic myeloid leukaemia
CNS	central nervous system
CRP	C-reactive protein
CT	computed tomography
D & C	dilatation and curettage
DRE	digital rectal examination
ENT	ears, nose, and throat
ESR	erythrocyte sedimentation rate
EVUS	endovaginal ultrasound
FAP	familial adenomatosis polyposis
FBC	full blood count
FOB	faecal occult blood
GGT	gamma glutamyl transferase
GI	gastrointestinal
HCG	human chorionic gonadotrophin
HNPCC	hereditary non-polyposis colorectal cancer
HPF	high-power field

HPV	human papillomavirus
HRT	hormone replacement therapy
HTLV	human T-cell lymphotrophic virus
IU	international unit
LDH	lactate dehydrogenase
LFT	liver function test
LHRH	luteinising hormone releasing hormone
LR	likelihood ratio
MGUS	monoclonal gammopathy of undetermined significance
MRI	magnetic resonance imaging
MSU	mid-stream urine
NMSC	non-melanocytic skin cancer
NRH	no rehydration
NSAIDs	non-steroidal anti-inflammatory drugs
NSCLC	non-small-cell lung cancer
OPD	outpatient department
PSA	prostate-specific antigen
RBC	red blood cell
RCT	randomised controlled trial
RH	rehydration
RR	relative risk
SCC	squamous-cell carcinoma
SCLC	small-cell lung cancer
SGOT	serum glutamic oxaloacetic transaminase
SIGN	Scottish Intercollegiate Guidelines Network
TNM	tumour, node, metastasis (classification system)
TRUS	transrectal ultrasonography
WBC	white blood cell

To Ailie, Emily, Siân, and Katrina

1

Introduction

As general practitioners, we seem to walk a tightrope, balancing the often-conflicting demands and expectations of patients, consultants, health authorities, or professional organisations. We are always concerned not to miss a serious or important condition in a patient, whereas, on the other hand, we are aware of the need to avoid overinvestigation or over-referral of patients. Such actions are both costly to the NHS as a whole and can have significant adverse consequences for individual patients.

In relation to cancer it is now known that one out of every 20 encounters with a GP will involve patients exhibiting one of the seven warning signals of cancer.[1] Moreover, in general, the earlier that a cancer is diagnosed, the better is the prognosis.

Five-year survival in early and late cancer

	Early (%)	Late (%)
Breast	75	<10
Colorectal	90	<30
Bladder	70	<30
Cervix	>75	5

This book seeks to fill a gap by acting as a concise, primary-care-based guide, which outlines epidemiological data, risk factors, symptoms, and signs of the more common cancers, along with the place and value of investigations. It is intended as an aid to clinical assessment and not a rigid or comprehensive textbook of oncology.

According to Morrell, GPs are primarily diagnosticians,[2] and yet it seems that diagnosis still remains the Achilles heel in general practice.[3] The problem is rooted in a misunderstanding of the differences between patients, pathologies, presentations, prevalences, and predictive values (the proportion of patients with a positive test result who have the target disorder) in hospital practice compared to primary care. It is self-evident that the spectrum of patients seen on a medical ward or in the surgical clinic differs considerably from that in primary care. What is less well appreciated is that as prevalences vary so will the predictive values of signs and symptoms (see Appendix 1).[4]

Within primary care, conditions will often be seen at an evolutionary stage when 'textbook' descriptions and classifications simply do not apply and sensitivities and specificities of features in the history, examination, or investigations are also changing. As will be seen in the discussion of lung cancer (Chapter 5), in the Papworth series, although cough was the most common complaint to the general practitioner, shoulder or chest pain was the initial complaint in one-third of patients, with only 3% presenting with haemoptysis.[5]

Decisions made by GPs are also different from those made by specialists – the precise diagnostic labels may be less important than deciding on an appropriate course of action. Diagnoses may be framed in terms of binary decisions: treatment versus non-treatment, referral versus non-referral, and serious versus not serious.[6] The information used to make such decisions may not only be the 'traditional' static clinical information but also information gained over a period of time (dynamic evidence) and clusters of information.

Certain pieces of clinical information more readily and uniquely available in primary care may have significant weights of evidence, assisting the diagnosis of malignancy in the primary-care setting. For example, over 30 years ago Pereira-Gray noted the importance of behaviour change in indicating a likelihood of malignancy;[7] one specific example often cited is a recent decision to stop smoking. In a large cohort study, Nylenna noted that the patient's fear of cancer was an important predictor of malignancy.[8] Olesen examined the pattern of attendance in patients for the 3 years prior to the diagnosis of cervical carcinoma and noted that significantly more patients than controls had had no doctor contact.[9]

In writing this book I have sought to collect, appraise, and summarise systematically all the available evidence relating to the identification of patients with the more common malignancies in a primary-care setting. Such identification may be by approaches that are either presymptomatic (e.g. breast cancer screening) or symptomatic (e.g. the rational approach to a patient aged 45 with rectal bleeding). Primary-care staff have a critical role in ensuring the success of population screening programmes for cancer.

Within each chapter, important diagnostic pointers in symptomatic patients may be found in the sections on epidemiology, risk factors, and anatomical distribution, as well as the symptoms, signs, and investigations. The assessment of the patient with potentially significant symptoms involves looking for features (or clusters of features) in the history, examination, or investigations to help us out of our uncertainty.

Sections have also been included in relation to some broader aspects of primary-care oncology, i.e. an overview of the pathology, prognosis, management, and follow-up after treatment. This serves to place the emphasis on early diagnosis in context and underlines the observation that it cannot be divorced from a broad understanding of treatment and prognosis. Twenty-five years ago, Howie pointed out that, as GPs, we often frame a diagnosis in terms of treatment options[10] – the observation that lung cancer is not universally fatal was an important lesson for myself in writing this book.

Some pieces of clinical information such as weight loss, back pain, or a raised erythrocyte sedimentation rate (ESR) are non-specific and, although they may, in certain circumstances, indicate a high probability of malignant disease, they do not fit neatly within a particular cancer. With this in mind, I have added a separate chapter focusing exclusively on such non-specific items of clinical information and their predictive values for the diagnosis of malignancy.

Advances in medical genetics have highlighted the value of family history taking. An average general practitioner would expect to have 30–40 patients on his list with a strong family history of cancer.[11] Such a history may increase their personal risk significantly and justify further action. Thus, in addition to specific sections in the chapters on colorectal cancer, breast cancer, and ovarian cancer, an overview of cancer genetics has been consolidated into a single chapter.

Although the search for evidence has been extensive (see Appendix 3 for the MEDLINE search strategy for ESR), it is clear that in many areas the primary-care evidence base remains unsatisfactory. This is certainly the case for cough and lung cancer[12] or haematuria and urological malignancies[13] in a primary-care setting. For the rarer cancers, the information presented within the chapters has necessarily been extracted from a broader range of sources, but it has been appraised and assembled from a primary-care clinical perspective. Hence, it is hoped that this book will also serve to emphasise the need for further rigorous epidemiological research into the diagnosis of cancer in primary-care settings.

References

1 Love N (1991) Why patients delay seeking care for cancer symptoms. What you can do about it. *Postgrad. Med.* **89**: 151–8.

2 Morrell DC (1993) *Diagnosis in general practice. Art or science?* Nuffield Provincial Hospitals Trust, London.

3 Howie JGR (1972) Diagnosis – the Achilles heel? *J. R. Coll. Gen. Pract.* **22**: 310–15.

4 Knottnerus JA (1991) Medical decision making by general practitioners and specialists. *Fam. Prac.* **8**: 305–7.

5 Varney VA, Atkinson TD, and Stark JE (1996) Lung cancer: importance of early signs. *Update* **57**: 120–5.

6 McWhinney IR (1997) *A textbook of family medicine.* Oxford University Press, Oxford.

7 Pereira-Gray DJ (1966) The role of the general practitioners in the early detection of malignant disease. *Trans. Hunterian Soc.* **25**: 135–79.

8 Nylenna M (1986) Diagnosing cancer in general practice: from suspicion to certainty. *BMJ* **293**: 314–17.

9 Olesen F (1988) Pattern of attendance at general practice in the years before the diagnosis of cervical cancer; a case control study. *Scand. J. Prim. Hlth Care* **6**: 199–203.

10 Howie JGR (1973) A new look at respiratory illness in general practice. *J. R. Coll. Gen. Pract.* **23**: 895–904.

11 Johnson N, Lancaster T, Fuller A, and Hodgson SV (1995) The prevalence of a family history of cancer in general practice. *Fam. Pract.* **12**: 287–9.

12 Liedekerken BMJ, Hoogendam A, Buntinx F *et al.* (1997) Prolonged cough and lung cancer: the need for more general practice research to inform clinical decision making. *Br. J. Gen. Pract.* **47**: 505.

13 Buntinx F and Wauters H (1997) The diagnostic value of macroscopic haematuria in diagnosing urological cancers: a meta-analysis. *Fam. Pract.* **14**: 63–8.

2

Some facts and figures

Overview

- Over 250 000 people in the UK develop cancer each year.
- There are over 200 different types of cancer, but just four types – lung, breast, colorectal, and prostate – account for half of all cases.
- Over 65% of all new cancers are diagnosed in people aged over 65 years.
- It is estimated that approximately 670 000 people in the UK are still alive following a diagnosis of cancer within the past 10 years.

Incidence

- The incidence refers to the number of new cases of cancer in a defined population during a specified time period.
- Numbers of new cancers registered in the UK during 1995:

Lung	40 260
Breast	33 240
Colorectal	31 230
Prostate	18 690
Oesophagogastric	17 020
Bladder	13 170
Non-Hodgkin's lymphoma	8240

Pancreas	6830
Ovary	5910
Leukaemias	5900
Kidney	5250
Melanoma	4980
Endometrial	4090
Brain	3910
Larynx/pharynx	3670
Cervix	3450
Myeloma	3450
Lip and mouth (oral)	2780
Testis	1380

Although the information available on the incidence of non-melanocytic cancers may be of lower quality, it is estimated that the incidence of such tumours amounts to 50 000 cases per annum in the UK.

- It is helpful to relate the incidence figures to an average list size for a general practitioner of approximately 2000 patients. Thus the impact on the 'average' general practitioner would be:

Skin	1 case every 6 months
Lung	1 case every 9 months
Breast	1 case every year
Colorectal	1 case every year
Prostate	1 case every 18 months
Oesophagogastric	1 case every 18 months
Bladder	1 case every 2 years
Non-Hodgkin's lymphoma	1 case every 3–4 years
Pancreas	1 case every 4 years
Ovary	1 case every 5 years
Leukaemias	1 case every 5 years
Kidney	1 case every 5 years
Endometrial	1 case every 7 years
Brain	1 case every 7 years
Larynx/pharynx	1 case every 8 years
Cervix	1 case every 8 years
Myeloma	1 case every 8 years
Lip and mouth (oral)	1 case every 10 years
Testis	1 case every 20 years

- The incidence of the most frequent forms of cancer vary by age.

Age (years)	Most common cancers (excluding non-melanocytic skin cancer)
0–14	Acute lymphoblastic leukaemia, central nervous system
15–29	Testis, cervix, Hodgkin's disease
30–54	Breast, lung
55–74	Lung, breast, colorectal, prostate

Prevalence

- The prevalence gives an indication of the numbers of people alive with cancer in a specified population at a designated time. Hence both the incidence and the longevity of individuals diagnosed with cancer influence the prevalence. Consequently, prevalence measures are most useful for healthcare providers, to assess the public health impact of a specific disease within a community and to project medical care needs for affected individuals
- Number of persons alive on 1 January 1991 diagnosed with cancer between 1981 and 1990 in England and Wales:

Breast	137 300
Colorectal (males and females)	80 200
Prostate	36 600
Bladder (males)	36 100
Lung (males and females)	28 500
Endometrial	21 500
Ovary	13 700

Further reading

Cancer Research Campaign (1998) *Incidence – UK.* Cancer Research Campaign: London.

Jones R and Menzies S (1999) *General Practice: Essential Facts.* Radcliffe Medical Press, Oxford.

3

Cancer genetics

Background

Epidemiology

- In a proportion of common cancers there may be a familial component.
- Of patients with breast, colon, or ovarian cancer, 5–10% will give a family history of relatives with the same cancer. Clearly some of these will be coincidental *but* others may reflect an inherited predisposition.
- About 1% of all cancers arise in individuals with an unmistakable hereditary cancer syndrome (e.g. familial adenomatomas polyposis, *see* Chapter 4).
- The average practitioner should expect to have 40–50 patients on his list with a strong family history of cancer.[1]
- There are interrelationships between different cancers: an inherited predisposition to one particular cancer may also increase the risk of developing other cancers.

Identifiable risk factors

There are a number of indicators of genetic predisposition to cancer:

- cancers with a familial component often present at a younger age (<50 years)
- multiple cancers in families (e.g. several cancers of the same type; 'associated' cancers in the family, i.e. breast, ovarian, bowel, or two or more cases of rare cancers)

- more than one primary tumour in an individual (e.g. bilateral breast cancer)
- in general terms, the following patients warrant further assessment:
  - patients in whose family there have been one or more cancers in first- or second-degree relatives under the age of 60
  - four or more relatives of any age with cancer.

Details of specific cancers are included in the appropriate chapters.

Molecular pathology

- Cancer is a gene-based disorder and is mediated by the activity of oncogenes and tumour-suppressor genes.

Examples of oncogenes associated with human cancers

Oncogene	Human cancer involvement	Protein properties
K-ras	Pancreatic, colorectal, lung (adenocarcinoma), endometrial	Regulation of intracellular signalling (p21 guanosine triphosphatase)
N-ras	Myeloid leukaemia	
H-ras	Bladder	
HST	Gastric	Growth factor
N-myc	Neuroblastoma, small-cell lung cancer	Transcription factor

Examples of tumour-suppressor genes associated with human cancers

Tumour-suppressor gene	Human cancer involvement	Function of protein product
TP53	Most common genetic change in cancers (inherited mutations in Li–Fraumeni syndrome)	Transcription factor
APC	Familial adenomatomas polyposis	Regulates B-catenin function
BRCA-1	Breast/ovarian	DNA repair
BRCA-2	Breast	

Figure 3.1 Cancer is a multistage process; for example, a number of stages have been suggested for colonic cancer.[2]

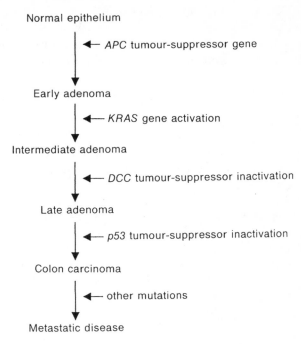

Normal epithelium

← *APC* tumour-suppressor gene

Early adenoma

← *KRAS* gene activation

Intermediate adenoma

← *DCC* tumour-suppressor inactivation

Late adenoma

← *p53* tumour-suppressor inactivation

Colon carcinoma

← other mutations

Metastatic disease

- Cancer is a multistage process. Although oncogenes and tumour-suppressor genes are essential for the evolution of human cancer, it is important to appreciate that, in general, a single gene will not cause cancer (Figure 3.1).
- At each stage the process can be seen in relation to Knudson's 'two hit' hypothesis. For example, for breast cancer, a woman with a germ-line alteration in one *BRCA-1* allele is born with a first 'hit' which increases her susceptibility to cancer. A second 'hit' must then inactivate the remaining normal allele for a clonal population of cancer cells to arise in the breast. This process takes a long time, about 15–20 years in the case of breast cancer.
- A number of factors may cause genetic changes involving the activation of oncogenes or the inactivation of tumour-suppressor genes.
  - hereditary factors (this chapter)
  - dietary factors, e.g. aflatoxin
  - smoking
  - viruses, e.g. human papillomavirus (HPV).

Cancer history taking in general practice

Traditionally, genetic counselling is best seen in terms of three elements – a diagnostic aspect (genetic assessment), the actual estimation of risks, and a supportive role ensuring that those given advice actually benefit from it and from the various management and preventative measures that may be available.

The diagnosis

- A clear diagnosis is an essential basis for accurate genetic counselling. Certainly, in relation to breast cancer, obtaining and interpreting an accurate and detailed family history remains the most important aspect of individual risk assessment. Unfortunately, family history taking is a neglected part of the assessment of patients in primary care.[3]
- Family history information must include:
  - details of cancers in as many maternal and paternal relatives as possible (NB the candidate breast cancer genes are not on the sex chromosomes); in any family history, distinction needs to be made between first- and second-degree relatives:
    - (i) first-degree relatives: mother, father, daughter, sister, brother, son
    - (ii) second-degree relatives: maternal grandparents, paternal grandparents, maternal aunts and uncles, paternal aunts and uncles
  - information on unaffected relatives must also be included since the distribution of unaffected and affected relatives within a family is essential for the assessment of inheritance patterns
  - information should be recorded for a minimum of three generations wherever possible and this may take a lot of time and correspondence
  - details such as age at diagnosis and age of unaffected individuals, tumour histology, the occurrence of bilateral tumours, and sites of primary tumours should be obtained wherever possible
  - it is also important to make a note of the presence of any genetic syndromes in the family, which might be associated with an increased risk of, for example, breast cancer.
- Clearly, there will be a number of difficulties in obtaining a reliable and clear diagnosis, e.g.
  - the affected individual may have lived a considerable time ago, when relevant diagnostic investigations were not available
  - the affected individual might have died without essential investiga-

tions having been done or without an autopsy having been performed
- a firm diagnosis cannot be reached even with the affected individual living
- the diagnosis may be wrong.

Practical considerations

- Taking a good family history is very time consuming (it is necessary to allow at least half an hour for an initial assessment in primary care).
- Nurses have been shown to be effective in compiling family histories as part of routine screening.
- Pedigree-drawing programmes are available on the Internet or in other published work (e.g. genograms).[4-6] An example of the form used by the Yorkshire Cancer Genetics Service is given in Figure 3.2.

The estimation of risks

- Once a reliable family history has been obtained, it is necessary to estimate the risk – this should be undertaken in consultation with published evidence (*see* chapters for each of the individual cancers) and local protocols. Occasionally special investigations can be utilised to alter the risk estimate.
- Any risk assessment should be carefully recorded and, in general practice, tagging the clinical records may be useful. Such tagging will enhance the ability to use the family history information in dealing with both symptomatic and asymptomatic patients.

The supportive role

Primary-care clinical staff will have an increasingly important role in this element of genetic counselling, especially for chronic diseases such as cancer. In particular it is important:
- to maintain up-to-date, reliable information on the current cancer genetic services and policies operational in your local area, including the feasibility and availability of genetic testing

Figure 3.2 Yorkshire Cancer Genetics Service cancer family history questionnaire. (Reproduced by kind permission of Dr Carol Chu.)

YORKSHIRE REGIONAL GENETICS SERVICE
DEPARTMENT OF CLINICAL GENETICS

PATIENT QUESTIONNAIRE REGARDING A FAMILY HISTORY OF CANCER

Most cancers arise by chance in an individual but in approximately 5% of people with certain types of cancer there may be an underlying genetic predisposition.

The Yorkshire Regional Genetics Service offers to see individuals with a family history of cancer to assess that individuals risks of developing cancer, suggest screening and offer tests if appropriate.

In order for us to be able to decide if there is a genetic predisposition in a family, it is extremely helpful for us to have details about the family history - particularly the type of cancers in the family and the age at which the individual developed the cancer.

Your doctor will give you this form to fill in and you can then send it to us when you have completed the details. We will assess your risks and then either suggest appropriate screening to your doctor, if this is necessary, or arrange to see you in one of our clinics.

PLEASE FILL IN YOUR DETAILS BELOW:

Name .... DOB ....

Address ....

.... Postcode .... Tel no: ....

G.P .... Referring Dr: ....

GP address ....

....

REFERRING DOCTORS COMMENTS:

Ashley Wing, St. James's University Hospital, Beckett St, Leeds LS9 7TF
Tel : 0113 206 6970/65927   Fax: 0113 246 7090

Please complete the form below, giving as much information as possible about your immediate (blood) relatives, **including** those who have not had cancer. If there is any information you do not know, perhaps someone in your family will be able to help you, otherwise leave that box empty. All the information you give will be held in confidence in the Clinical Genetics Unit.

RELATIVE	NAME (INCLUDING MAIDEN AND ANY PREVIOUS NAMES)	DATE OF BIRTH	ALIVE YES/NO	DATE OF DEATH	IF YOUR RELATIVE SUFFERED FROM CANCER...			
					TYPE OF CANCER	AGE AT DIAGNOSIS * MOST IMPORTANT	SMOKE YES / NO	HOSPITALS WHERE TREATED
SELF								
YOUR OWN CHILDREN								
YOUR SISTERS FULL OR HALF (ie share one parent)								
YOUR BROTHERS FULL OR HALF (ie share one parent)								
YOUR MOTHER								
YOUR MOTHER'S MOTHER								

| RELATIVE | NAME (INCLUDING MAIDEN AND ANY PREVIOUS NAMES) AND ADDRESS | DATE OF BIRTH | ALIVE YES/NO | DATE OF DEATH | IF YOUR RELATIVE SUFFERED FROM CANCER... | | | |
					TYPE OF CANCER	AGE AT DIAGNOSIS * MOST IMPORTANT	SMOKE YES / NO	HOSPITALS WHERE TREATED
YOUR MOTHER'S FATHER								
YOUR MOTHER'S BROTHERS & SISTERS								
YOUR FATHER								
YOUR FATHER'S MOTHER								
YOUR FATHER'S FATHER								
YOUR FATHER'S BROTHERS & SISTERS								
ANY OTHER RELATIVES WITH CANCER (PLEASE SPECIFY RELATIONSHIP)								

Ethnic origin   Eastern European / Jewish / Asian / Afro-Carribean
Other (please specify)

Date: /   /19

- to convey to individuals, especially those at low risk, accurate information in a sensitive and supportive manner
- to refer individuals where the genetic risk is likely to be high, to the specialist cancer genetics team
- to provide ongoing support for individuals who are significantly distressed by their cancer family history and to refer them to specialist help if necessary
- to form a partnership with the specialist cancer genetics clinics, cancer centres, and cancer units to ensure that referral guidelines are locally appropriate and that education material is relevant for all members of the primary healthcare team.

Genetic testing for cancer

- There is a current vogue for genetic testing in cancer, even to the extent of screening.[7–9]
- Genetic testing is a time-consuming process. The first step is to identify the faulty gene in the family and then to offer genetic testing to unaffected individuals in that family.
- As with any proposed screening test, it is necessary to consider other features, e.g. the natural history and the potential for treatment of the condition or abnormality identified.
- Even in families with a large number of relatives affected with breast or ovarian cancer, the unaffected individuals still have at least a 50% chance of inheriting the 'good' copy of the gene.
- Individual patients often have little understanding of possible inherited predispositions in relation to cancer and may opt for such testing without being adequately informed.

Methods of genetic testing

- There are two stages in the identification of a cancer-predisposing gene: linkage mapping and isolation of the gene itself. Genetic testing can be done at either stage.
- Linked markers depend on their physical proximity on the chromosome to the 'cancer gene'. For general population screening it is essential to identify the predisposing 'cancer gene' itself.
- For any genetic test, blood must be obtained from a consenting affected relative.

Genetic testing for BRCA-1[10,11]

- *BRCA-1* is a long gene with 100 000 base pairs.
- Mutations in this gene are typically said to be associated with an extremely high lifetime risk of cancer of the breast (87%) and ovaries (44%).
- These mutations account for an estimated 10–30% of all women diagnosed with breast cancer under the age of 45. However, from a public-health perspective, this only amounts to 5% of breast cancer patients overall.
- To date, more than 100 variants of *BRCA-1* have been shown to be associated with tumour growth.
- *BRCA-1* is only the first of a number of genes involved in inherited breast cancer.
- The quality of some genetic tests for *BRCA-1* may not be satisfactory – present techniques probably only detect 80% of such mutations (the figure has been placed as low as 60%). It is also very difficult to discriminate between disease-associated mis-sense variants and 'polymorphic' variants.

The link to the phenotype

- Uncertainty about who will develop disease is an inherent part of genetic testing.
- The multistage nature of cancer, variable expressivity, incomplete penetrance, and genetic heterogeneity all reduce the ability of genetic tests to predict future disease accurately, even when single genes have a prominent role.
- The fact that a woman from a 'cancer-prone' family tests positive for one of the cancer-linked DNA variants does not mean that she will have a tumour, even though her lifetime risk of breast cancer may be as high as 85% (although it does seem that even this risk may be an overestimate due to the effects of multiple genetic alterations and multiple modifiers).
- Communicating such uncertainty to patients may be very difficult. Better ways to help clinicians communicate probabilities to patients are needed.

When to test

- There is great uncertainty about the right time in a person's life to perform a test.

Treatment options

- Although treatments are available for some of the common complex disorders, such as breast (*see* Chapter 6) and colon (*see* Chapter 4) cancer, their safety and effectiveness in asymptomatic people found to have genetic susceptibilities to these disorders have not been established. Prophyactic mastectomy remains controversial.[12]
- Surveillance methods continue to evolve and require evaluation.[13,14]
- It is difficult to know what other lifetime or preventative modifications should occur once a test has been reported.

Social implications[15-17]

- Test results can have adverse consequences for the psychological well-being, family relationships, employability and insurability of those tested.
- According to Giardiello *et al.*,[18] patients who underwent genetic testing for familial adenomatous polyposis often received inadequate counselling and incorrectly interpreted results.

Key point

Genetic testing is best sought from specialised centres in which the indicators for such tests and their results can be interpreted, patient's confidentiality is maintained, and psychosocial support is available for patients and family members.

Somatic mutations in cancer diagnosis: the future

- As indicated earlier, only a small fraction of all cancers arise in individuals who carry a germline defect conferring genetic predisposition.
- Many genes underlying inherited cancer syndromes have more widespread roles in sporadic cancers, as a result of somatic mutations that arise during tumour initiation and progression.
- Identification of such somatic mutations by molecules in, for example, urine, blood, or stool may have implications for both the early diagnosis and the early diagnosis of recurrence for a number of cancers.[19]

Tumour	Somatic mutation detected
Bladder cancer diagnosis	Urinary *p53*, chromosome 9 (short arm detection)
Colorectal cancer diagnosis	Blood/stool K-*ras* and *p53* genes

- The molecular assessment of cancer may also become of increasing importance in relation to staging, prognosis, and in guiding treatment.

Further reading

Gogas H and Sacks NPM (1996) Familial breast cancer. *Cancer J.* **9**: 115–17.
Harper PS (1993) *Practical genetic counselling.* Butterworth-Heinemann, Oxford.
Lynch HT, Fusaro RM, and Lynch J (1995) Hereditary cancer in adults. *Cancer Detect. Prevent.* **19**: 219–33.
Report of a Working Group for the Chief Medical Officer (1996) *Genetics and Cancer Services.* Department of Health, London.

References

1 Johnson N, Lancaster T, Fuller A, and Hodgson SV (1995) The prevalence of a family history of cancer in general practice. *Fam. Pract.* **12**: 287–9.
2 Haber DA and Fearon ER (1998) The promise of cancer genetics. *Lancet* **351** (Suppl. II): 1–8.
3 Summerton N and Garrood PVA (1997) The family history in family practice: a questionnaire study. *Fam. Pract.* **14**: 285–8.
4 Progeny at http:/tprogeny2000.com/body.shtml
5 Jameson MJ (1968) A system of recording the family history in general practice. *J. R. Coll. Gen. Pract.* **16**: 135–43.
6 Jolly W, Froom J, and Rosen MG (1980) The genogram. *J. Fam. Pract.* **10**: 251–5.
7 Rahman MI, Dennis LK, and Gibson-Sheve LD (1997) Selections from the current literature: issues in genetic testing for cancer. *Fam. Pract.* **14**: 510–16.
8 Welch HG and Burke W (1998) Uncertainties in genetic testing for chronic disease. *JAMA* **280**: 1525–7.
9 Olopade OI (1996) Genetics in clinical cancer care – the future is now. *NEJM* **335**: 1455–6.
10 Lerman C, Narod S, Schulman K *et al.* (1996) BRCA-1 testing in families with hereditary breast–ovarian cancer. A prospective study of patient decision making and outcomes. *JAMA* **275**: 1885–92.

11 Couch FJ and Hartman LC (1998) BRCA-1 testing – advances and retreats. *JAMA* **279**: 955–7.

12 Fentiman I (1998) Prophylactic mastectomy: deliverance or delusion? *BMJ* **317**: 1402–3.

13 Burke W, Petersen G, Lynch P *et al.* (1997) Recommendations for follow-up care of individuals with an inherited predisposition to cancer. I. Hereditary nonpolyposis colon cancer. *JAMA* **277**: 915–19.

14 Mackay J (1998) Introducing a cancer genetics service: oncologists invited to comment. *Cancer Top.* **10**: 1–3.

15 Marteau TM and Croyle RT (1998) Psychological responses to genetic testing. *BMJ* **316**: 693–6.

16 Holtzman NA and Shapiro D (1998) Genetic testing and public policy. *BMJ* **316**: 852–6.

17 Geller G, Botkin JR, Green MJ *et al.* (1997) Genetic testing for susceptibility to adult-onset cancer. The process and content of informed consent. *JAMA* **277**: 1467–74.

18 Giardiello FM, Brensinger JD, Pedersen GM *et al.* (1997) The use and interpretation of commercial APC gene testing for familial adenomatous polyposis. *NEJM* **336**: 823–7.

19 Caldas C (1998) The molecular assessment of cancer. *BMJ* **316**: 1360–3.

4

Colorectal cancer

Background

Epidemiology

- In 1995 31 250 individuals were diagnosed with colorectal cancer in the UK. This amounts to just over one new case per GP per year.
- The incidence of colorectal cancer rises rapidly after the age of 50:

Age	Age-standardised rates/100 000 individuals/annum
<50 years	4
50–69 years	100
Over age 70	300

- Colorectal cancer is recognised as a disease of economically developed countries.

Identifiable risk factors

Extremely high risk

- Familial adenomatosis polyposis (FAP) – estimated to account for 1% of new cases of colorectal cancer.

- Hereditary non-polyposis colorectal cancer (HNPCC) – estimated to account for 5% of new cases of colorectal cancer.
- Long-standing (>10 years) and extensive ulcerative colitis – estimated to account for 1% of new cases of colorectal cancer.

Moderately increased risk (2–3 times normal)

- Personal history of colorectal cancer or adenomas.
- Positive family history but no identifiable syndrome (*see* below).

Colorectal cancer genetics

- Colorectal cancer has a large familial component: it has been estimated that a quarter of new colorectal cancers may arise in individuals with an inherited genetic predisposition.
- Two genetic syndromes are of particular importance:
  - familial adenomatosis polyposis (FAP):
    (i)   accounts for 1% of all new colorectal cancers
    (ii) caused by mutations in the tumour-suppressor gene 'adenomatosis polyposis coli' (*APC*) on chromosome 5
    (iii) autosomal dominant
    (iv) new mutations of the *APC* gene are not uncommon and about 30% of cases actually have no family history of colorectal cancer
    (v)   clear phenotype: multiple colorectal adenomas develop during childhood/adolescence, progressing to adenocarcinomas by the age of 40
    (vi) all affected individuals will develop colon cancer if the colon is left *in situ*
    (vii) extracolonic features include pigmented lesions of the fundus, osteomas, and epidermoid cysts.
  - hereditary non-polyposis colorectal cancer (HNPCC):
    (i)   accounts for 5% of all new colorectal cancers
    (ii) autosomal dominant, caused by mutation in the mismatch repair genes
    (iii) there is no clear phenotype
    (iv) the lifetime risk of developing bowel cancer is approximately 80% (especially right-sided colorectal cancer)
    (v)   it has an early onset (average age at diagnosis = 45 yrs)
    (vi) it is associated with an increased risk for other cancers, e.g. endometrial, ovary, stomach, urinary tract, small bowel and biliary tract).
- Familial clustering: aside from the syndromes, close relatives of people diagnosed with colorectal cancer are at increased risk.

- In assessing risks for an individual patient, account needs to be taken of both the numbers of first-degree relatives affected and their ages at diagnosis.
- It is important to stress that only family histories which consist of an early onset relative (under the age of 45) or many affected relatives are associated with significantly increased risks in relatives.

Overall the following patients warrant further assessment (greater than 10% lifetime risk):

(i) one first-degree relative affected, diagnosed with colorectal cancer before the age of 45

(ii) at least two first-degree relatives of any age affected with colon cancer

(iii) families with at least two individuals with colorectal cancer, plus endometrial, ovarian, stomach, urinary tract, biliary tract or small bowel cancers (i.e. evidence of a dominant family cancer trait).

- **Please check on the local approach recommended in your area.**

Anatomical distribution of tumours (incidence data)

Caecum/ascending colon	15%
Sigmoid region	40%
Rectum	35%

Pathology and prognosis

The mortality of colorectal cancer is closely linked to the stage at diagnosis:

Dukes' stage (modified)	Definition	Approximate frequency at diagnosis (%)	Five-year survival (%)
A	Cancer localised within the bowel wall	11	83
B	Cancer which penetrates the bowel	35	64
C	Cancer spread to lymph nodes	26	38
D	Cancer with distant metastasis (most often in the liver)	29	3

Treatment overview

- As surgery remains the mainstay of treatment and offers the best chance of permanent cure, all patients with suspected colorectal cancer should be referred for appropriately informed surgical opinion.
- Certain categories of patient (e.g. Dukes' B and C colorectal tumours) may subsequently be considered for adjuvant chemotherapy and/or radiotherapy.
- For primary-care practitioners, three important factors need to be borne in mind:
  - The long-term results of surgery remain disappointing. This is mainly due to the late and advanced presentation of over one-quarter of colorectal cancers. There is some evidence that a reduction in the time between the onset of symptoms and referral to hospital results in an improvement in the Dukes' staging.[1]
  - Of patients with colorectal cancers, 20–30% present as emergencies with intestinal obstruction or, occasionally, perforation or bleeding. Such patients are invariably older and frailer than average: the mortality in this group is considerably increased (postoperative mortality 19% compared to 8% in comparable elective cases). It has been suggested that such cases represent a marker for failure of adequate diagnostic assessment within primary care.[2]
  - There are usually significant delays from the onset of symptoms to surgical treatment. Such delay can occur at three different levels: delay on the part of the patient, delay by the general practitioner prior to patient referral, and delay incurred at the hospital after patient referral. Macadam reported a range in patient delay from 1 week to 2 years.[3] Reasons given by patients for delay include fear, ignorance about the significance of symptoms, or simply being oblivious to symptoms. Only a small proportion of individuals regularly look at their stools or at the toilet paper on defecation.[4]

Screening for colorectal cancer

Family history

- It has been suggested that invasive screening (i.e. colonoscopy, double-contrast barium enema, and sigmoidoscopy) should be offered to all first-degree relatives of patients with FAP or HNPCC. According to guidelines produced by the Scottish Intercollegiate Guidelines Network (SIGN) such investigations should be commenced in the teens when

FAP is diagnosed and approximately 10 years later in the case of HNPCC. The recommended screening interval is 1–3 years.

- It has been recommended that all patients with a greater than a 10% lifetime risk of colorectal cancer (*see* p. 25) warrant further assessment. The following approach has been suggested:[5]
  - invasive screening should be targeted on younger people at high risk
  - persons with a family history who are not from families with HNPCC/FAP should be offered faecal occult blood testing at age 40.
- **It is important to check on the local approach adopted in your area**, i.e. to enquire about the type of screening recommended for the various 'at-risk' populations, the age at which such screening should commence, and the chosen screening interval. It is also helpful to be aware of the preferred management options available locally.

Faecal occult blood testing

- Faecal occult blood (FOB) tests detect the peroxidase-like activity of haemoglobin in the stools and rely on the tendency of colorectal cancers to bleed.
- In the Nottingham trial, the sensitivity was 74% and the specificity 98%.[6] However, in the Danish trial, the sensitivity was lower at 48% (specificity 99%).[7]
- Sensitivity is limited because may cancers and polyps bleed intermittently, so that blood is unevenly distributed in the faeces.
- Rehydration (RH) of the slide increases the sensitivity at the expense of specificity.[8] In one study, sensitivity increased from 57.9% to 78.9% whereas specificity decreased from 96.6% to 93.8% with rehydration (i.e. fewer false negatives but more false positives).[9]
- Randomised controlled trials (RCTs) have shown that population screening (average-risk individuals) for colorectal cancer with FOB tests can reduce mortality from colorectal cancer by 15–32%. The details of the trials are illustrated in the table overleaf.
- A recent meta-analysis of the studies from Minnesota, Nottingham, and Denmark, together with a further study from Sweden, concluded that:
  - screening reduced mortality from colorectal cancer by 16% for those allocated to screening and by 23% for those who were actually screened
  - a biennial haemoccult screening programme offered to 10 000 people aged greater than 40 years (of whom about two-thirds attended for at least one test) should prevent 8.5 deaths from colorectal cancer over 10 years.[10]
- **The number needed to screen** is defined as the number of people that

	University of Minnesota[8]	Nottingham study[6]	Danish study[7]
Year began	1975	1981	1985
No. of subjects	46 000	152 850	137 485
Age (years)	50–80	45–74	45–75
Method	RH	NRH	NRH
Compliance (%)	77	59.6	67
Decrease in death rates between groups from cancer (%)	32	15	18

NRH, no rehydration.

need to be screened for a given duration to prevent one death or one adverse event. For haemoccult screening this figure can be calculated to be 1274 for 5 years (compared with 2451 for women aged 50–59 screened by mammography).[11]

Colorectal cancer screening with faecal blood testing: overview

The disease	Response	Comment
Is it an important problem?	Yes	see p. 23
Is the natural history well understood?	Reasonably but not fully understood	
Is there a recognised latent or early stage?	Yes	Generally accepted that most cancers arise from adenomatous polyps

The test – faecal occult blood testing	Response	Comment
Is it simple to perform?	Reasonably	See below
Is it expensive?	No	These factors
Is it sufficiently accurate?	Sensitivity (NRH) has been estimated to be 48% and 74% in trials	will be evaluated formally in the
Is it acceptable with adequate compliance?	59.6% compliance in UK trial[7]	colorectal cancer national screening pilots[12]

Are there adequate facilities for the diagnosis and treatment of any abnormalities detected?	The standard follow-up for people with positive tests is colonoscopy, with double-contrast barium enema for those for whom a complete colonoscopy cannot be carried out. Another option is to offer a combination of double-contrast barium enema and sigmoidoscopy	See above

The treatment	*Response*
Is there any effective treatment?	Yes
Does treatment at an earlier stage result in more benefit than treatment started at a later stage?	Yes (the RCTs addressed this question)

Practical considerations

Guidelines for FOB testing (reproduced with permission, based on work by Dr H. Griffiths, Consultant Chemical Pathologist, Huddersfield):

- Patients must have an appropriate diet before the test. The most important dietary advice is (1) to eat a diet high in roughage for 3 days before and during the test period, and (2) not to take any vitamin C supplements, which may cause negative interference.
- In some other testing methods it is also necessary to avoid red meat, cauliflower, and broccoli.
- Aspirin, non-steroidal anti-inflammatory drugs (NSAIDs), and iron tablets do not interfere significantly.
- The test envelopes may have a limited shelf-life. Some laboratories prefer to supply plastic stool-collection pots to GPs rather than test envelopes themselves. **Please check on your local arrangements**.

In the forthcoming colorectal cancer national screening pilots it is proposed that the following process should be followed:[12]

- biennial screening using the FOB test between ages 50 and 69 years
- a reminder letter after 4 weeks to those who have not responded

- no rehydration of samples
- no dietary restrictions
- the FOB test consists of a specially treated paper cut into six squares:

Result	Action
5/6 positive squares	Referral for further investigation
1/4 positive squares	Repeat test after restricting meat intake in diet

Flexible sigmoidoscopy

- Although the results of two ongoing RCTs are not yet available, case-control studies suggest that sigmoidoscopy can reduce mortality from colon cancers.
- In a recent study comparing flexible sigmoidoscopy with FOB screening in primary care it was concluded that:
  - flexible sigmoidoscopy detects more adenomas and cancer than screening with a FOB test
  - high uptake of flexible sigmoidoscopy screening is achievable provided accurate call-up lists are used.[13]

Symptoms in primary-care

- Symptoms pointing to a possibility of colorectal cancer can be divided into:
  - bleeding symptoms (e.g. anaemia, rectal bleeding)
  - abdominal symptoms (e.g. change in bowel habit, abdominal pain)
  - systemic symptoms (e.g. unexplained weight loss, general malaise, and tiredness).
- A number of studies have indicated that rectal bleeding is not uncommon in the general population (20% per year)[14] and yet only 1 out of 25 people with rectal bleeding consults the GP for this complaint. This represents an 'iceberg phenomenon'.
- Following this selection by the patients, a second filtration takes place in general practice, with 7% of all patients with rectal bleeding being referred on for further assessment.[15] Slight changes in bowel habit are also relatively common in the general population and go through a similar selective process.[16]
- Although the risk of colorectal cancer increases with age, a significantly

higher proportion of elderly people report symptoms attributable to the lower gastrointestinal (GI) tract.[17]

- It is important to:
  - encourage patients with 'significant symptoms' to consult the general practitioner promptly (*see* below); patients may ignore, not notice, or fail to appreciate the significance of important symptoms – in the assessment of any bowel or abdominal symptom it is important to enquire specifically about rectal bleeding
  - ensure that the 'right' patients are being referred on for appropriate assessment.
- Research in primary-care populations indicates that the following are the most important individual symptoms:
  - change in bowel habit (for greater than 2 weeks)
  - blood or mucus seen mixed or on the stool
  - abdominal pain
  - unexplained weight loss
  - general malaise and tiredness, e.g. related to anaemia.
- In view of the prevalence of these symptoms in the normal general population, it is often more valuable to think in terms of 'symptom clusters'. Research indicates that combinations of bleeding symptoms and of abdominal symptoms are particularly valuable in pointing the way to a need for further, urgent action.

Bleeding symptoms

- **Age greater than 50, change in bowel habit (for greater than 2 weeks), blood seen mixed or on the stool**.[18,19] A study by Norrelund and Norrelund suggests that, as well as a first bleeding episode, similar importance should be attached to a change in a known bleeding pattern.[20]
- **Age greater than 50, change in bowel habit (for greater than 2 weeks), positive faecal occult blood**.[21] According to Leicester *et al.*, haemoccult has a high specificity for colorectal cancer in symptomatic patients (84.5%). Thus in accord with the rule of SpPin (*see* Appendix 1: 'if a test has sufficiently high specificity, a positive result rules in the disorder'), FOB testing may be useful in adding further evidence to a diagnostic problem. However, in view of the lower sensitivity (the FOB test fails to detect 20–50% of cancers and up to 80% of polyps), a negative result cannot be used in symptomatic patients to rule out colorectal cancer.[22]
- **Patients with unexplained iron deficiency anaemia and change in bowel habit**. Patients with iron-deficiency anaemia over the age of 45 should be fully investigated for gastrointestinal cancer by upper and

lower GI endoscopy (*see also* Chapter 13). In a recent audit of 109 cases of iron-deficiency anaemia presenting to a single district laboratory, 19% had investigation of both the upper and lower gastrointestinal tract, 21% the upper gastrointestinal tract only and 7% the lower gastrointestinal tract only. In 55 cases no endoscopic or radiological investigation was performed. Eighteen months after presentation, nine colorectal cancers, five gastric cancers, and 11 peptic ulcers had been diagnosed; 21 patients had died, including two from colorectal cancers not detected when the iron-deficiency anaemia presented.[23]

Abdominal symptoms

- In a general practice population with non-acute abdominal complaints, some clinical findings can be used as independent predictors for neoplastic gastrointestinal disease – male sex, greater age, no specific character to pain, weight loss, and ESR greater than 20 mm/h.[24] These individual items of information can be built into 'clusters' with powerful predictive value:

	Probability for neoplastic disease (%)
Age > 65, male	3
Age > 65, male, non-specific abdominal pain	18
Age > 65, male, non-specific abdominal pain and weight loss	50
Age > 65, male, non-specific abdominal pain, weight loss, and ESR > 20 mm/h	75

- **Differentiation from irritable bowel syndrome** can be very difficult. However, a number of studies have confirmed that the following symptoms are more common in irritable bowel syndrome than in other gastrointestinal diseases considered to be organic:
  - pain relief with bowel action
  - more frequent stools with the onset of pain
  - looser stools with the onset of pain
  - passage of mucus
  - sensation of incomplete evacuation
  - abdominal distension as evidenced by tight clothing or visible appearance.

Among 60-year-old women, 80% had irritable bowel syndrome when all six symptoms were present compared with only 38% when two symptoms were present. However, it is important to appreciate that the predictive ability of the six criteria diminishes with increasing age and the criteria are less useful in men than in women.[25]

Signs: the examination

- Rectal examination remains a neglected part of the assessment of patients with symptoms pointing towards the possibility of colorectal cancer.[26]
- MacArthur and Smith reported that patients who were not given a rectal examination at their first consultation experienced considerably more delay in being referred for specialist opinion.[27]
- Digital rectal examination can reach 15–30% of colorectal tumours, most rectal carcinomas and rectal polyps.[28] A rectal examination can also detect altered bowel contents in terms of blood or mucus on the examining finger.
- Other significant clinical findings are infrequent but consist of abdominal tenderness and/or mass.

Practical considerations

Guidelines for rectal examination (reproduced with permission, based on work by Mr R. Goodall, Consultant Surgeon, Halifax):
- **When to?** With the probable exception of children and patients with a fissure, any patient with anorectal symptoms must have a rectal examination performed, if only to help assess urgency of referral.
- **Position?** The patient should be in the left lateral position with spine flexed. It helps if his or her head is to the far edge of the couch and hips on the near side.
- **Inspection?** Look at the perineum as well as the anal area. If the skin is sore or if there are ulcers, fistulas, prolapsed or thrombosed haemorrhoids, then extra care is needed to prevent a painful examination. Remember that gentle traction on the perianal skin may reveal a fissure, in which case it is best not to proceed with a digital examination. Refer urgently to the outpatient department for treatment.
- **Palpation?** With plenty of lubricant on the gloved index finger, place the palmar aspect of the tip to the anus. Apply firm but gentle pressure until the sphincter relaxes. Only then insert the finger into the anal canal. If there is no relaxation and there is pain, think 'fissure'. Poster-

iorly, the sacrum and coccyx will be felt; anteriorly the prostate will be felt in males and the cervix uteri in females. Unless they are thrombosed, internal haemorrhoids are **not** palpable. Therefore any other mass is **abnormal** and potentially sinister. Remember to examine the glove after withdrawal. The presence of mucus and/or blood and the stool colour are all important. Finally, remove any excess lubricant from the perianal skin.

Radiological investigations and local referral patterns

- In suspected cases of colorectal cancer, the large bowel can be completely examined by one of two methods: colonoscopy or sigmoidoscopy plus double-contrast barium enema. **It is important to check on the local referral patterns and arrangements in your area.**
- Any investigation, either radiological or laboratory based, should only be undertaken if the practitioner considers that the outcome of that investigation will materially affect his or her decision. As with any investigation there may be false negatives. In situations where the history and examination indicate a high likelihood of colorectal cancer (e.g. change in bowel habit, rectal bleeding and age over 50) it may be more appropriate to arrange a direct referral to an appropriate colorectal surgeon.
- Local cancer units and centres should adhere to quality criteria in order to minimise unnecessary delays in diagnosis and treatment.

Follow-up and detection of recurrence

- Follow-up may include any combination of the following, carried out at intervals ranging from every 3 months to yearly: clinical examination, colonoscopy, barium enema, sigmoidoscopy, FOB tests, serum carcinoembryonic antigen (CEA) tests, computed tomography (CT) scan, chest radiography, full blood count, liver function tests, and hepatic imaging.
- Although CEA testing can sometimes permit earlier detection of recurrence, it seems that most patients with rising CEA have other symptoms anyway, e.g. a change in bowel habit or bleeding.
- Three recently published randomised controlled trials have compared regular follow-up with no follow-up, or 'conventional' with 'intensified' protocols. An overview of the three concluded that none showed any significant variation in outcome (5-year survival).

- Although it has been suggested that regular specialist follow-up may offer patients support and reassurance, it is clear that some patients may be falsely reassured and delay seeking help for significant symptoms by waiting for the next follow-up appointment. It seems that the majority of recurrences produce symptoms between follow-up appointments.
- Patients with colorectal cancer are at risk of developing further carcinomas in the residual colon and rectum (metachronous tumours). As a consequence some have advocated regular colonoscopic surveillance, but a recent trial concluded that yearly colonoscopy (combined with liver CT and chest radiography) did not improve survival when added to symptom and simple screening review.[29]

General sources of information

NHS Centre for Reviews and Dissemination, University of York (1997) *Effective Health Care Bulletin: The Management of Colorectal Cancer*. FT Healthcare, York.

NHS Executive Guidance on Commissioning Cancer Services (1997) *Improving Outcomes in Colorectal Cancer. The Manual and Research Evidence*. Department of Health, London.

Scottish Intercollegiate Guidelines Network (SIGN) (1997) *Colorectal Cancer*. SIGN publication No. 16. SIGN, Edinburgh.

References

1 Robinson M, Thomas W, Hardcastle JD *et al.* (1993) Change towards earlier stage at presentation of colorectal cancer. *Br. J. Surg.* **80**: 1610–12.

2 Hargarten SW, Roberts MJS, and Anderson AJ (1992) Cancer presentation in the emergency department: a failure of primary care. *Am. J. Emerg. Med.* **10**: 290–3.

3 Macadam D (1979) A study in general practice of the symptoms and delay patterns in the diagnosis of gastrointestinal cancer. *J. R. Coll. Gen. Pract.* **29**: 723–9.

4 Carter S and Winslet M (1998) Delay in the presentation of colorectal cancer: a review of causation. *Int. J. Colorect. Dis.* **13**: 27–31.

5 Dunlop M and Campbell H (1997) Screening for people with a family history of colorectal cancer. *BMJ* **314**: 1779–80.

6 Hardcastle JD, Chamberlain JO, Robinson MHE *et al.* (1996) Randomised controlled trial of faecal-occult-blood screening for colorectal cancer. *Lancet* **348**: 1472–7.

7 Kronborg O, Fenger C, Olsen J *et al.* (1996) Randomised study of screening for colorectal cancer with faecal-occult-blood test. *Lancet* **348**: 1467–71.

8 Mandel JS, Bond JH, Church TR *et al.* (1993) Reducing mortality from colorectal cancer by screening for fecal occult blood. *NEJM* **328**: 1365–71.

9 Walter SD, Frommer DJ, and Cook RJ (1991) The estimation of sensitivity and specificity in colorectal cancer screening methods. *Cancer Detect. Prevent.* **15**: 465–9.

10 Towler B, Irwig L, Glasziou P *et al.* (1998) A systematic review of the effects of screening for colorectal cancer using the faecal occult blood test, Hemoccult. *BMJ* **317**: 559–65.

11 Rembold CM (1998) Number needed to screen: development of a statistic for disease screening. *BMJ* **317** 307–12.

12 National Screening Committee (1998) *A Proposal for Colorectal Cancer Screening Pilots.* Department of Health, London.

13 Verne JECW, Aubrey R, Love SB *et al.* (1998) Population based randomised study of uptake and yield of screening by flexible sigmoidoscopy compared with screening by faecal occult blood testing. *BMJ* **317**: 182–5.

14 Crosland A and Jones R (1995) Rectal bleeding: prevalence and consultation behaviour. *BMJ* **311**: 486–8.

15 Thompson M and Prytherch D (1996) Rectal bleeding: when is it right to refer? *Practitioner* **240**: 198–200.

16 Jones ISC (1976) An analysis of bowel habit and its significance in the diagnosis of carcinoma of the colon. *Am. J. Proct.* **45**: 45–56.

17 Curless R, French J, Williams GV, and James OFW (1994) Comparison of gastrointestinal symptoms in colorectal carcinoma patients and community controls with respect to age. *Gut* **35**: 1267–70.

18 Fijten GH, Starmans R, Muris JWM *et al.* (1995) Predictive value of signs and symptoms for colorectal cancer in patients with rectal bleeding in general practice. *Fam. Pract.* **12**: 279–86.

19 Helfand M, Marton KI, Zimmer-Gembeck M, and Sox HC (1997) History of visible rectal bleeding in a primary care population. Initial assessment and 10-year follow-up. *JAMA* **277**: 44–8.

20 Norrelund N and Norrelund H (1996) Colorectal cancer and polyps in patients aged 40 years and over who consult a GP with rectal bleeding. *Fam. Pract.* **13**: 160–5.

21 Holtedahl KA (1989) *Diagnosis of cancer in general practice.* MD Thesis, University of Tromso.

22 Leicester RJ, Lightfoot A, Millar J *et al.* (1983) Accuracy and value of the Hemoccult test in symptomatic patients. *BMJ* **286**: 673–4.

23 Lucas CA, Logan ECM, and Logan RFA (1996) Audit of the investigation and outcome of iron-deficiency anaemia in one health district. *J. R. Coll. Phys. Lond.* **30**: 33–5.

24 Muris JWM, Starmans R, Fijten GH *et al.* (1995) Non-acute abdominal complaints in general practice: diagnostic value of signs and symptoms. *Br. J. Gen. Pract.* **45**: 313–16.

25 Lynn RB and Friedman LS (1995) Irritable bowel syndrome. *Med. Clin. North Am.* **79**: 373–90.

26 Hennigan TW, Franks PJ, Hocken DB, and Allen-Mersh TG (1990) Rectal examination in general practice. *BMJ* **301**: 478–80.

27 MacArthur C and Smith A (1983) Delay in the diagnosis of colorectal cancer. *J. R. Coll. Gen. Pract.* **33**: 159–61.

28 Umpleby HC, Bristol JB, Rainey JB, and Williamson RCN (1984) Survival of 727 patients with single carcinomas of the large bowel. *Dis. Colon Rectum* **27**: 803–10.

29 Schoemaker D, Black R, Giles L, and Toouli J (1998) Yearly colonoscopy, liver CT, and chest radiography do not influence 5-year survival of colorectal cancer patients. *Gastroenterology* **114**: 7–14.

5

Lung cancer

Background

Epidemiology

- Lung cancer developed in just over 40 000 individuals in the UK during 1995. Some 39 000 died of the disease in 1992. This amounts to over one new case per GP per year. It is the most frequent cancer that a GP will encounter.
- Lung cancer is the most common type of cancer in men and the second most common type of cancer in women.
- Lung cancer is rare under the age of 40.

Major identifiable risk factors

- Smoking: 90% of lung cancer deaths in the UK are attributed to smoking. The highest risks appear to be associated with heavy and persistent year-on-year cigarette smoking. Overall the risk of lung cancer in a smoker is 15 times that of a non-smoker. Although the risk of coronary heart disease quickly subsides after giving up smoking, the risk of lung cancer remains throughout life.
- Recently evidence has been produced that passive smoking is also a risk for lung cancer.[1] It is estimated that at least 300 people die each year in the UK from lung cancer caused by passive smoking.

Other risk factors

- Radon gas (estimated to cause 5% of lung cancer deaths).
- Asbestos (estimated to cause 2% of lung cancer deaths).

Anatomical distribution

Seventy-five per cent of tumours arise in the main bronchi; the remainder are peripheral.

Pathology and prognosis

- Pathological types:

Small-cell (SCLC) (oat cell)	25%
Non-small cell (NSCLC)	
squamous carcinomas	50%
adenocarcinomas	15%
large-cell carcinomas	10%

- International TNM (tumour, node, metastasis) staging system for lung cancer:

Stage		Five-year survival (%)
I	Small tumour, no nodes or metastasis	60–80
II	Small tumour, nodes but not mediastinal nodes; no metastasis	25–40
III(a)	Large tumour, ipsilateral mediastinal nodes are present; no metastasis	10–30
III(b)	Contralateral mediastinal or any scalene or supraclavicular nodes; no metastasis	<5
IV	Metastatic disease	<5

- Lung cancer is potentially curable but overall the prognosis of all lung cancer remains poor – 80% die within a year of diagnosis and only 5.5% survive 5 years.
- In view of the effect of stage on survival, it is clear that primary-care clinicians have an important role in ensuring early diagnosis and rapid referral of patients with symptoms and signs suggestive of possible lung cancer to an appropriate specialist service.
- Currently, there is a mean delay of 7 months between the initial presentation of symptoms in primary care and ordering a chest radio-

graph. Consequently, 80–90% of NSCLC patients present late with unresectable disease (stage III/IV). Only 10–20% present with stage I and II disease.

- Patients with disease not amenable to radical therapy have a median survival of 6 months or less. Only about 5% of SCLC patients survive 5 years, compared with 10–20% of those with NSCLC. SCLC generally has the worst overall survival because of its frequent and more rapid spread to the mediastinum and major organs.
- Earlier diagnosis also serves to ensure that palliative care services for the patient can be better planned and delivered at an earlier stage.

Treatment overview

- **SCLC**: the first-line treatment for SCLC is normally chemotherapy (supplemented, when appropriate, with radiotherapy). With chemotherapy, the median survival of patients with limited disease is between 10 and 16 months.
- **NSCLC**: Where appropriate, surgery may offer the hope of cure in NSCLC. NSCLCs are usually slower growing than SCLC. Fitter individuals with early-stage cancers, which can be treated by surgery, have a much better prognosis.

Screening for lung cancer

- A recent systematic review of screening for lung cancer (by chest radiography and/or sputum cytology) concluded that routine screening for lung cancer among asymptomatic people is not effective.[2]
- The potential screening tools, sputum cytology and/or chest radiographs, have high false-negative rates, high follow-up testing requirements and low yields.
- In the three main randomised controlled trials conducted in the 1970s (Mayo Clinic, Johns Hopkins, and Memorial–Sloane Kettering hospitals), involving 30 000 male smokers over the age of 45, there was no evidence that such screening reduced long-term mortality, despite the finding that initially more cases of early-stage lung cancer were detected in the screened group, with improved 5-year survival (lead-time and length-time bias – see Appendix 1).[3]
- Occasionally smokers attend the surgery for reassurance and a 'check up'. In such patients two factors should be borne in mind:
  - The average, asymptomatic, middle-aged smoker walking into the GPs surgery actually has a low probability of lung cancer (most

likely less than 1%, i.e. the likelihood of 'no disease' is 99% or greater). Assuming (generously) that a routine chest radiogram has a sensitivity of 50%, then it is important to appreciate that the 'new likelihood for no disease' after performing the chest radiogram will only have increased to a maximum of 99.5%. It is therefore very important not to falsely reassure such patients.

- Primary-care clinicians can be effective in promoting smoking cessation. We need to identify systematically all tobacco users at every visit and strongly urge and assist them to quit. The table below lists three effective interventions to help people stop smoking.[4]

Type of intervention	Quit rate
Brief advice from health professionals	2%
Nicotine replacement plus advice, support, or counselling	12%
10 minutes' (minimum) prenatal counselling for pregnant women, plus written material tailored to pregnancy	15%

Symptoms in primary care

- **Chronic cough and lung cancer**: the frequency of cough in patients with newly diagnosed lung cancer varies between 21% and 87%, but chronic cough ultimately occurs in up to 90% of lung cancer patients. However, although chronic cough (lasting longer than 3 weeks) may be one of the most important features of early lung cancer, the diagnostic value of a single finding of prolonged cough for lung cancer in a non-referred primary-care setting remains uncertain.[5]
- **The differential diagnosis** of chronic cough is extensive; the common causes of chronic cough are listed below. According to O'Connell, the greatest diagnostic challenge is presented by the persistent dry cough.[10]

Setting	Community[6]	Referral[7]	Consecutive, referral[8]	Consecutive, referral[9]
Benchmark	Retrospective review, including response to treatment	Chest X-ray plus response to treatment	Questionnaire chest X-ray plus response to treatment	Questionnaire respiratory function tests, plus response to treatment
Eligible/followed up	134/139	49/?	88/98	45/61
Asthma (%)	21	24	14	29
Postnasal drip (%)	19	41	38	56
Acid reflux (%)	4	21	40	11
Postinfectious (%)	9	–	–	–
Chronic bronchitis bronchiectasis (%)	4	5	4	–
Other (%)	–	–	8	4
Undiagnosed (%)	14		2	

- **Papworth series**: a retrospective study of the case histories of 316 patients with primary lung cancer attending Papworth Hospital revealed the following:[11]

Initial complaint to GP	Number (%) of patients
Cough	117 (37%)
Shoulder/chest pain	104 (33%)
Breathlessness	35 (11%)
Weight loss with malaise	17 (5%)
Haemoptysis	10 (3%)
Hoarseness	9 (3%)

The most common first symptom was either cough or localised chest or shoulder pain. In 80% of patients the cough was a new symptom, in 20% a previous cough had changed in character. Similar results were obtained in a small Swedish study, with cough, dyspnoea, and chest pain being the most frequent initial symptoms.[12]

- **Philadelphia Pulmonary Neoplasm Research Project**: from 1951, 6027 men aged 45 or older were screened radiologically every 6 months for 10 years and questioned about symptoms and smoking habits.[13] They were self-selected volunteers and some were lost to follow-up. The risk of lung cancer according to the clinical features were as follows:

Clinical feature	Risk of lung cancer (%)
Lung fields clear on chest radiograph on entry to study and asymptomatic	1.78
Lung fields unclear on chest radiograph on entry to study (i.e. non-specific lung disease)	2.64
Chronic cough	2.98
Hoarseness	3.42
Coughing smokers (i.e. more than 1 pack/day for 40 years)	8.81

- In a study from a specialised setting, 'chronic cough' had a high negative (0.99) and a low positive predictive value (0.03), i.e. the absence of a cough is helpful in excluding lung cancer whereas the presence of a cough is unhelpful in diagnosing lung cancer.[14]
- Clusters of clinical information may be helpful (e.g. age, sex, symptoms, and history of smoking). In the age groups 60–69 years, the likelihood ratios (LRs) are as follows:[15]

Clinical information	LR for lung cancer in males/females 60–69 years	
	Male	Female
Hoarseness or coughing without any apparent reason and non-smoker	19	8
Hoarseness or coughing without any apparent reason and smoker	52	50

- Significance should be attached to persistent and resistant chest infections (*see* p. 46).

Signs: the examination

- Examination by the general practitioner is often quite normal. In the small Swedish study, no abnormal signs were found in over a quarter of the patients.[12]
- The presence of any persistent localised chest sign (e.g. signs of lung collapse, consolidation, respiratory noises, or pleural effusion) in a smoker warrants further investigation.
- Clubbing and hypertrophic pulmonary osteoarthropathy occur in 2–12% of patients with lung cancer (most commonly NSCLC). With the decline in the incidence of chronic pulmonary infectious diseases,

carcinoma of the lung is the leading cause of hypertrophic osteoarthropathy.
- Metastatic disease is most likely to affect the brain, liver, and bones.
- Determining whether patients with lung cancer have metastatic disease
  is crucial to optimum management. A meta-analysis by Silvestri *et al.*
  revealed that clinical assessment was very powerful in screening for
  metastatic disease (negative predictive value greater than 97%).[16]

Clinical findings suggesting metastatic disease

- Symptoms elicited in history:
    - constitutional: weight loss greater than 10 pounds (4.5 kg)
    - musculoskeletal: focal skeletal pain
    - neurological: headaches, syncope, seizures, extremity weakness,
      recent change in mental status.
- Signs found on physical examination:
    - lymphadenopathy (greater than 1 cm)
    - hoarseness, superior vena cava syndrome
    - bone tenderness
    - hepatomegaly (greater than 13 cm)
    - focal neurological signs, papilloedema
    - soft-tissue mass.
- Routine laboratory tests:
    - hematocrit, less than 40% in males
    - hematocrit, less than 35% in females
    - abnormal liver function tests (elevated alkaline phosphatase, GGT or
      ALT).

A negative clinical evaluation based on these criteria should reassure the
clinician that the likelihood of obtaining a positive brain or abdominal CT
or radionuclide bone scan is small.

Investigations

- The aims of investigations are to:
    - confirm the presence of lung cancer
    - to determine the tumour type.
  Such information is essential for decision making about management.
- Patients with symptoms or signs suggestive of lung cancer should be
  referred to a chest physician.
- An urgent chest radiogram usually assists with the diagnosis **but**, as
  with any investigation, there may be false negatives. If the history,

symptoms, and signs are suggestive of early lung cancer, a negative chest radiogram should not alter the referral decision.

- Haemoptysis, hoarseness, or localised persistent chest signs require referral for bronchoscopy even in the absence of abnormalities on a chest radiogram.
- The median time for radiological resolution after community-acquired pneumonia is 6 weeks. This needs to be borne in mind when following up such patients.
- There is no role for sputum cytology examination, in view of its low sensitivity. Although tumour type can sometimes be identified from sputum cytology, this method cannot be used to exclude lung cancer because it has a high false negative rate.
- Spirometry: in view of the close relationship between lung cancer and diseases characterised by airflow obstruction, it has been suggested that airflow obstruction could be a strong indicator of the presence or likelihood of cancer.[17]
- In the small Swedish study, the most common abnormal laboratory finding was a raised ESR (>30 mm/h).[12] For further information on the ESR, *see* Chapter 18.

Solitary pulmonary nodule

Occasionally a solitary pulmonary nodule is found on a chest radiogram taken for unrelated reasons. The evidence indicates that:

- about 40% of solitary pulmonary nodules reported in various series are malignant
- the likelihood of malignancy depends on the patient's age, smoking history and the lesion's size and appearance
- lesions that have central calcifications on chest radiograms or have been stable for more than 2 years are usually benign.[18]

Follow-up and detection of recurrence

- According to Walsh *et al.*, screening for asymptomatic recurrences in patients who have had lung cancer is unlikely to be cost effective. Frequent follow-up and extensive radiological evaluation of patients after operation for lung cancer is probably unnecessary.[19] As a result of their study, they recommended the following follow-up procedure:
  - for the first year postoperatively, the patient should have physician or nurse practitioner contact, with chest radiography every 6 months
  - after the first year, chest radiography should be performed annually,

with other radiological evaluations only in patients in whom symptoms develop.

It is important to check on the local follow-up arrangements operating in your area.

Local referral patterns

- Open-access chest radiography referral is now generally available, and the reporting is subject to regular audit.
- Patients with suspected lung cancer should be referred to an appropriate chest physician urgently. It is often possible to phone the consultant's secretary and arrange for the patient to be seen prior to the next bronchoscopy list.
- There should be a clear, district-based clinical policy, which describes the pathway of care for the diagnosis of lung cancer. It is essential to check the local arrangements operating in your area.
- Local cancer units and centres should adhere to quality criteria in order to minimise unnecessary delays. Ideally no more than 6 weeks should elapse between GP presentation with suspicion of lung cancer and histological diagnosis.

General sources of information

Feld R, Ginsberg RJ, Payne DG, and Shepherd FA (1995) Lung. In: MD Abeloff, JO Armitage, AS Lichter, and JE Niederhuber (eds) *Clinical Oncology*. Churchill-Livingstone, New York.

NHS Centre for Reviews and Dissemination, University of York (1998) *Effective Health Care Bulletin: The Management of Lung Cancer*. FT Healthcare, York.

NHS Executive Guidance on Commissioning Cancer Services (1998) *Improving Outcomes in Lung Cancer. The Manual and Research Evidence*. Department of Health, London.

Scottish Intercollegiate Guidelines Network (SIGN) (1998) *Management of Lung Cancer*. SIGN publication No. 23. SIGN, Edinburgh.

References

1   Barnes DE and Bero LA (1998) Why review articles on the health effects of passive smoking reach different conclusions. *JAMA* **279**: 1566–70.
2   Wolpaw DR (1996) Early detection in lung cancer. *Med. Clin. North Am.* **80**: 63–82.
3   George PJM (1997) Delays in the management of lung cancer. *Thorax* **52**: 107–8.

4   Agency for Health Care Policy and Research (1996) *Smoking Cessation*. Clinical Practice Guideline No. 17. AHCPR, Rockville.

5   Liedekerken BMJ, Hoogendam A, Buntinx F *et al*. (1997) Prolonged cough and lung cancer: the need for more general practice research to inform clinical decision-making. *Br. J. Gen. Pract.* **47**: 505.

6   Poe RH, Harder RV, Israel RH, and Kallay MC (1989) Chronic persistent cough: experience in diagnosis and outcome using an anatomic diagnostic protocol. *Chest* **95**: 723–8.

7   Irwin RS, Corrao WM, and Pratter MR (1981) Chronic persistent cough in the adult: the spectrum and frequency of causes and successful outcome of specific therapy. *Am. Rev. Respir. Dis.* **123**: 413–17.

8   Mello CJ, Irwin RS, and Curley FJ (1996) Predictive values of the character, timing and complications of chronic cough in diagnosing its cause. *Arch. Intern. Med.* **156**: 997–1003.

9   Pratter MR, Bartter T, Akers S, and DuBois J (1993) An algorithmic approach to chronic cough. *Ann. Intern. Med.* **119**: 977–83.

10   O'Connell F (1998) Management of persistent dry cough. *Thorax* **53**: 737.

11   Varney VA, Atkinson TD, and Stark JE (1996) Lung cancer: importance of early signs. *Update* **57**: 120–5.

12   Mansson J and Bengtsson C (1994) Pulmonary cancer from the general practitioner's point of view. *Scand. J. Prim. Hlth Care.* **12**: 39–43.

13   Boucot KR, Seidman H, and Weiss W (1977) The Philadelphia pulmonary neoplasm research project. *Envir. Res.* **13**: 451–69.

14   Patrick H and Patrick F (1995) Chronic cough. *Med. Clin. North Am.* **79**: 361–72.

15   Holtedahl KA (1989) *Diagnosis of cancer in general practice*. MD Thesis, University of Tromso.

16   Silvestri GA, Littenberg B, and Colice GL (1995) The clinical evaluation for detecting metastatic lung cancer. A meta-analysis. *Am. J. Respir. Crit. Care Med.* **152**: 225–30.

17   Petty TL (1995) Let's identify lung cancer early. *Chest* **108**: 887–8.

18   Tape TG (1991) Solitary pulmonary nodule. In: RJ Panzer, ER Black, and P. Griner (eds) *Diagnostic Strategies for Common Medical Problems*. ACP, Philadelphia.

19   Walsh GL, O'Connor M, Willis KM *et al*. (1995) Is follow-up of lung cancer patients after resection medically indicated and cost-effective? *Ann. Thorac. Surg.* **60**: 1563–72.

6

Breast cancer

Background

Epidemiology

- There were just over 33 000 new cases of breast cancer in 1995.
- Breast cancer causes 13 000 deaths per annum in England and Wales.
- Breast cancer is the leading cause of death in women aged 35–54 and the most common cause of cancer death amongst all women.
- The incidence is particularly high in Caucasian women over the age of 50.
- Breast cancer is more common in women of higher rather than lower socio-economic status.
- There is considerable geographical variation in the incidence of breast cancer around the world (i.e. North America and northern Europe have a higher incidence than Africa or Asia). Individuals migrating from areas of low incidence to areas of high incidence will assume the same risk as those in their new environment (e.g. Japanese migrants to the USA).
- Male breast cancer is rare, occurring 100 times less frequently than in women. It presents at an older age, on average in the mid-sixties.

Identifiable risk factors

- Younger age at menarche (a girl having menarche at age 12 has a 20% greater risk than a girl does with a menarche at age 16).

- Menopause after 55 years (twice the risk of women having menopause before the age of 45).
- Pregnancy: nulliparity and delayed birth of first child until after the age of 35 years (twice the risk of women having their first child before age of 20).
- Oral contraceptives: when the overall risk of breast cancer amongst users of oral contraceptive has been studied in large populations, no increased risk of breast cancer has been seen. However, there is a general consensus from studies in younger women that a small, but measurable, risk of breast cancer induction exists for women who use such contraceptives at a young age, especially before their first pregnancy. It is important to consider this in context, especially in relation to the protective effect against ovarian cancer, *see* Chapter 10.
- Hormone replacement therapy (HRT): over a large number of studies, the excess risk for users of postmenopausal HRT is approximately 10–40%. This risk appears to dissipate quickly after oestrogen use is discontinued.
- Previous history of breast cancer (lifelong risk of recurrence, especially in first few years after diagnosis).
- Increasing age (breast cancer is rare in women under 30, but the risk rises steadily with age).
- Previous irradiation to the breast.
- Benign breast disease:
  - slightly increased risk (1.5–2 times): palpable cysts
  - moderately increased risk (4–5 times): atypical hyperplasia.
  This risk is increased further if there is a positive family history.
- Family history: of the known risk factors for breast cancer, a positive family history is one of the most important (present in 5% of cases).

Breast cancer genetics

- Over one-quarter of the younger patients with breast cancer have a strong family history.
- The extent of the risk is dependent on:
  - the number and relationships of relatives affected
  - the age of onset of disease
  - the presence or absence of bilateral primary cancers
  - the presence or absence of multiple primaries at any site.
- BRCA-1/BRCA-2 genes increase susceptibility to breast cancer. They are located on chromosome 17 and confer an increased lifetime risk of breast cancer of up to 80–90% (*see* Chapter 3).

- According to Mackay, it is possible to stratify those presenting with a family history of breast cancer into three groups, high risk, moderate risk, and low risk:[1]
  - high-risk patients, who require referral to the cancer genetic clinic or the consultant in cancer genetics:
  (i)   breast or breast and ovarian families with four or more relatives affected at any age
  (ii) breast cancer only families with three relatives affected under 40
  (iii) breast and ovarian cancer families with three relatives affected; average age of breast cancers under 60
  (iv) families with one member with both breast and ovarian cancer.
  - moderate-risk patients need to be discussed with the local breast surgical team for consideration for regular mammography screening:
  (i)   one first-degree female relative with breast cancer under 40.
  (ii) one second-degree paternal female relative with breast cancer under 40
  (iii) one first-degree female relative with bilateral breast cancer under age 60
  (iv) two first- or second-degree female relatives with breast cancer under the age of 60 or ovarian cancer at any age
  (v)   three first- or second-degree female relatives with breast or ovarian cancer
  (vi) one first-degree male relative with breast cancer.
  - **Please check on the local approach recommended in your area.**

Anatomical distribution

Most carcinomas arise in the upper outer quadrant of the breast and are solitary.

Pathology and prognosis

- Breast cancer types: the classification is complex but virtually all are adenocarcinoma and the majority (80%) are ductal.
- Breast cancer has a long natural history.
- Clinical staging and prognosis:

Stage		Five-year survival (%)
I	Breast lump smaller than 2cm with no evidence of spread	84

II	Breast lump and palpable axillary lymph nodes	71
III	Tumour large and fixed to chest wall	48
IV	Distant metastasis present	18

- The TNM staging system is the most frequently used system to guide both treatment and prognosis. In operable cases, the 5- and 10-year survivals are approximately 80% and 60% for node-negative patients, 60% and 40% for node-positive patients.
- In assessing prognosis and diagnostic delay, a consistent and direct relationship was found between delay and tumour size, nodal involvement, presence of metastasis, and histological grade of disease at diagnosis.[2]
- Diagnostic delay has been attributed to the patient in two-thirds of cases and to the doctor in one-third of cases.[3,4]

Treatment overview

- Surgery, e.g. breast-conserving surgery such as lumpectomy plus radiotherapy or mastectomy.
- Adjuvant systemic therapy using tamoxifen, ovarian ablation or chemotherapy improves survival and recurrence rates.[5]

Effects of approximately 5 years of tamoxifen on mortality among women with a hormone-sensitive breast cancer

	Ten-year mortality among 1000 women
Breast cancer	~ 80 fewer
Endometrial cancer	~ 2 more
Pulmonary embolus	~ 1 more
Other causes of death	No difference
Overall effect on death: ~ 30 times more good than harm	

- The choice of adjuvant systemic therapy is influenced by a number of considerations, in particular:
  - the patient's age
  - the characteristics of the tumour.

Breast screening

- Randomised trials have shown that breast screening can reduce mortality from breast cancer by 17–31%. The details of three of the earlier trials are illustrated below.

	HIP[6]	Ostergotland[7]	Edinburgh[8]
Age group (years)	40–64	40–74	45–64
Screening method	Clinical and two-view mammography	One-view mammography	Clinical and mammography two-view initially, one-view on follow-up
Screening interval (years)	1	1.5–3	2
Reduction in mortality (%)	30 (after 10 years)	31 (after 7 years)	17 (after 7 years)

- An overview of all of the Swedish randomised controlled trials (Malmo, Kopparberg, Ostergotland, Stockholm, and Gothenburg) revealed a 24% significant reduction of breast cancer mortality among those invited to mammography compared with those not invited after 5–13 years of follow-up.[9]
- In the UK, breast screening by mammography is currently offered to all women aged 50–64 every 3 years. Women aged 65 and over may be screened on request.
- The standard screening technique used in the NHS Breast Screening Programme from March 1988 was the single mediolateral oblique view. In December 1994 it was agreed that a second (craniocaudal) view should be taken at a woman's first screening appointment. The decision stemmed from concerns about the number of cancers presenting during the interval between the 3-yearly screening appointments.
- Based on current evidence, asymptomatic referral to the screening programme is **not** routinely recommended for women under 50.
- It has been suggested recently that the upper age for screening should be raised to 69 years and the screening interval should be decreased to 2 years.
- A recent review of the value of breast examination by health professionals as a screening tool concluded that there was no evidence in support of its efficacy. There is a risk of giving false reassurance to women.[10]
- The effectiveness of breast self-examination in reducing mortality

from breast cancer has never been consistently demonstrated. In addition, it produces a high number of false positives and can cause unnecessary anxiety. In 1991 it was recommended that breast self-examination should no longer be promoted; instead women should become 'breast aware'. The concept of breast awareness is now widely accepted and women should be encouraged to be familiar with the feel and look of their breasts throughout the menstrual cycle.[11]

Breast screening with mammography: overview

The disease	Response	Comment
Is it an important problem?	Yes	See p. 49
Is the natural history well understood? (In order to determine screening interval)	Reasonably,	but there are variations in growth rates and metastatic potential
Is there a recognised latent or early stage?	Yes	Small cancers (<2 cm) are less likely to have metastasised

The test – mammography	Response	Comment
Is it simple to perform?	No	Equipment and staff
Is it expensive?	Yes	Equipment and staff
Is it sufficiently accurate?	Reasonable	Sensitivity approaches 85–90%; the two-view method is more accurate
Is it acceptable with adequate compliance?	Reasonable	Some concerns about discomfort anxiety and radiation risk. In the pilot the compliance was 64% so primary-care staff need to encourage uptake
Are there adequate facilities for the diagnosis and treatment of any abnormalities detected?	Yes	Established as part of the programme by the Forrest Report[12]

The treatment	Response
Is there any effective treatment?	Yes
Does treatment at an earlier stage result in more benefit than treatment started at a later stage?	Yes (the RCTs addressed this question, although the initial results from the Edinburgh study were not statistically significant)

- The uptake of mammography amongst the eligible population is a very important determinant of the effectiveness of the breast-screening programme.
- The attitudes of general practitioners and other primary-care staff to breast screening are critical in influencing women to attend screening.
- General practitioners and practice nurses have an important role in providing information, advice, and reassurance to women at all stages of the screening process.

Symptoms in primary care

Symptoms pointing to the possibility of breast cancer can be divided into five main groups:
- New lump or mass (three-quarters of patients); may be discrete or in a pre-existing nodularity.
- Nipple discharge in the over-50s or persistent bloodstained discharge in younger patients (sufficient to stain clothes).
- Nipple retraction, distortion, or an eczema-like rash.
- Breast contour change.
- Intractable or unilateral pain (rare).
- **Clearly a quarter of patients may present with symptoms other than lumps**. These patients unfortunately often suffer the longest delays and the worst outcomes.

Signs: the examination

- Ninety per cent of lumps are noted by women themselves.
- Clinical examination should be proficient and not delegated to staff who are not appropriately trained.

- It should involve examination of both breasts and axillae and, if necessary, examination of other areas.
- Premenopausal women are best examined 1 week after the onset of the last menstrual period, when engorgement of the breast is at a minimum.
- If a lump is detected, certain features of the lump increase the chance that it will be malignant:[13]

Breast mass characteristic	Sensitivity for cancer (%)	Specificity for cancer (%)	Likelihood ratio for cancer
Not soft or cystic	62	90	6.2
Irregular borders	60	90	6.0
Not freely moveable	40	90	4.0

- Clinical examination is not completely reliable:
  - in mammographic screening 60% of carcinomas detected are impalpable; most doctors cannot palpate a mass smaller than 8–10 mm, so nearly all very early lesions will be found by mammography
  - clinical examination has a sensitivity of 86% in detecting breast lumps (but may be as low as 37% in women under the age of 35)
  - the error rate in the clinical assessment of axillary lymph node metastases is between 30 and 50%
  - the golden rule is to 'pursue every breast complaint to resolution'.
- The approach to lumps and nipple discharge is detailed in Figures 6.1 and 6.2.[14]

Investigations

- Mammography has a sensitivity of 85–90% for the diagnosis of breast cancer.
- False negatives are more likely to occur in the following groups of patients. Those with:
  - breast pain
  - nipple discharge
  - nipple scaling
  - breast inflammation
  - breast mass or thickening in women with dense breasts
  - younger patients.
- It is important to consider referral of any women with suspicious signs or symptoms, irrespective of the result of a recent mammogram.
- All diagnostic modalities have an error rate and it is advisable to use

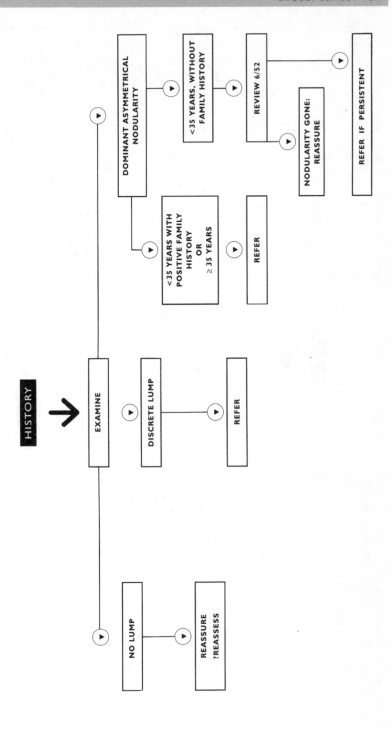

Figure 6.1 Guidelines for referral of patients with breast lumps. (Reproduced with permission of Dr Joan Austoker, CRC Primary Care Education Research Group.)

Figure 6.2 Guidelines for referral of patients with nipple discharge. (Reproduced with permission of Dr Joan Austoker, CRC Primary Care Education Research Group.)

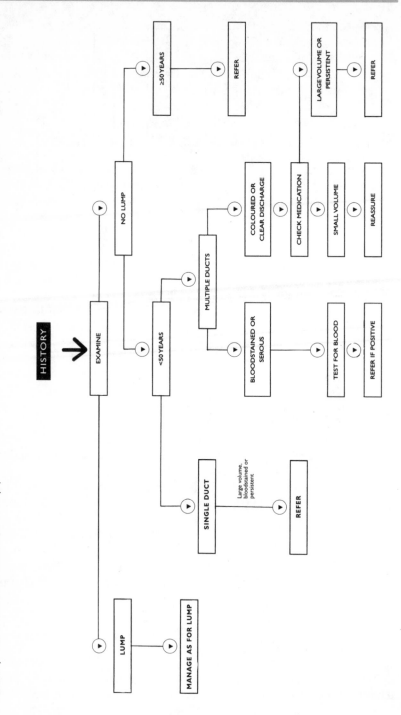

more than one modality to obtain a preoperative diagnosis. This is the approach used in breast clinics. The combination of clinical examination, mammography, ultrasonography, and fine-needle aspiration cytology provides the highest diagnostic accuracy and the lowest risk of diagnostic error (especially in women over the age of 35).

Follow-up and detection of recurrence[15,16]

- Recurrence is highest in the first years after surgery – regular mammography (yearly for the first 5 years after surgery and then 2-yearly) is recommended in order to detect local recurrence or a second primary in the contralateral breast. It is important to check on local arrangements.
- There is good evidence from two RCTs in Italy that intensive follow-up (i.e. hospital physician visits, bone scans, sonograms, chest radiographs, laboratory testing together with mammography) is not associated with better 5-year survival than normal follow-up.
- In the UK primary-care-based follow-up has been shown to be acceptable to patients and general practitioners. General-practitioner follow-up was not associated with increased time to diagnosis or increase in patient anxiety.
- Most recurrences are detected by women as interval events and present to the GP irrespective of continuing hospital follow-up.
- If follow-up is to take place in primary care, the following points need to be borne in mind:
  - the frequency of any visits must be adjusted to the patient's needs
  - some women at increased risk of relapse (e.g. those aged under 35) may still best be served by hospital follow-up
  - physical examination should include breasts, regional lymph nodes, chest wall and abdomen; the arms should be examined for lymphoedema
  - in women who are taking tamoxifen, it is important to enquire about vaginal bleeding (*see* p. 52)
  - patients should always be encouraged to report new persistent symptoms promptly without waiting for the next scheduled appointment.

Local referral patterns

- There is good evidence that the survival of patients with breast cancer is better if they are treated by a specialist who also treats a large number of similar patients in a multidisciplinary setting; GPs need to be aware of this in making appropriate referrals.

● Urgent referrals should be seen urgently. There is evidence that patient anxiety is less when they receive services promptly. Local cancer centres and units should adhere to quality criteria in order to minimise unnecessary delays.

● Many areas have rapid-access breast clinic services. It is essential to check on the local arrangements operating in your area.

General sources of information

Cancer Research Campaign (1996) *Breast Cancer – UK*. Cancer Research Campaign, London.

Cancer Research Campaign (1997) *Breast Cancer Screening*. Cancer Research Campaign, London.

Dixon M and Sainsbury R (1993) *Handbook of Diseases of the Breast*. Churchill Livingstone, London.

NHS Centre for Reviews and Dissemination, University of York (1996) *Effective Health Care Bulletin: The Management of Primary Breast Cancer*. FT Healthcare, York.

NHS Executive Guidance on Commissioning Cancer Services (1997) *Improving Outcomes in Breast Cancer. The Manual and Research Evidence*. Department of Health, London.

Silverstein MJ (1997) Diagnosis and treatment of early breast cancer. *BMJ* **314**: 1736–9.

References

1 Mackay J (1998) Introducing a cancer genetics service: oncologists invited to comment. *Cancer Topics* **10**: 1–3.

2 Osuch JR and Bonham VL (1994) The timely diagnosis of breast cancer. *Cancer* **74**: 271–8.

3 Rossi S, Cinini C, Pietro CD *et al.* (1990) Diagnostic delay in breast cancer: correlation with disease stage and prognosis. *Tumori* **76**: 559–62.

4 Burgess CC, Ramirez AJ, Richards MA, and Love SB (1998) Who and what influences delayed presentation in breast cancer? *Br. J. Cancer* **77**: 1343–8.

5 Early Breast Cancer Trialists' Collaborative Group (1998) Tamoxifen for early breast cancer: an overview of the randomised trials. *Lancet* **351**: 1451–67.

6 Shapiro S, Venet W, Strax P *et al.* (1982) Ten to fourteen-year effect of breast cancer screening on mortality. *J. Nat. Cancer Inst.* **69**: 349–55.

7 Tabar L, Fagerberg CJD, Gad A *et al.* (1985) Reduction in mortality from breast cancer after mass screening with mammography. *Lancet* **I**: 829–32.

8 Roberts M, Alexander FE, Anderson TJ *et al.* (1990) Edinburgh trial of screening for breast cancer: mortality at 7 years. *Lancet* **I**: 241–6.

9   Nystrom L, Rutqvist LE, Wall S *et al.* (1993) Breast cancer screening with mammography: overview of Swedish randomised trials. *Lancet* **341**: 973–8.

10   Department of Health (1998) Clinical examination of the breast. Professional Letter: PL/CMO/98/1. Department of Health, London.

11   Department of Health (1991) Breast awareness. Professional Letter: PL/CMO/91/15. Department of Health, London.

12   Department of Health and Social Security Working Group on Breast Cancer Screening (1986) *Breast Cancer Screening: Report to the Health Ministers of England, Wales, Scotland and Northern Ireland* (The Forrest Report). HMSO, London.

13   Mushlin AI (1991) Breast cancer. In: RJ Panzer, ER Black, and P Griner (eds). *Diagnostic Strategies for Common Medical Problems*. ACP, Philadelphia.

14   Austoker J, Mansel R, Baum M *et al.* (1999) *Guidelines for Referral of Patients with Breast Problems*. NHS Breast Screening Programme, Sheffield.

15   Grunfeld E, Mant D, Yudkin P *et al.* (1996) Routine follow up of breast cancer in primary care: randomised trial. *BMJ* **313**: 665–9.

16   Grunfeld E, Mant D, Vessey MP, Yudkin P (1995) Evaluating primary care follow-up of breast cancer: methods and preliminary results of three studies. *Ann. Onc.* **6**: S47–S52.

7

Prostate cancer

Background

Epidemiology

- In 1995 there were 18 690 new cases of prostate cancer in the UK.
- In British men prostate cancer is the third most common cause of cancer death, with 8689 deaths in 1993.
- The incidence of prostate cancer increases with age: only 12% of clinically apparent cases arise before the age of 65.
- The prevalence of prostate cancer is 36 600 (*see* Chapter 2).

Identifiable risk factors

- Genetic susceptibility in younger patients (family history of prostate cancer and/or breast cancer in first-degree relatives). It has been estimated that 43% of cancers diagnosed under the age of 55 years have an inherited risk, falling to 9% of cases diagnosed over the age of 80.
- Dietary factors: high saturated fat intake is associated with an increased risk.
- Occupational risk: radiation, cadmium.

Anatomical distribution

The prostate gland can be divided into three anatomical zones. In general, the majority of cancers occur in the peripheral parts of the prostate whereas in benign enlargement the transitional zone is more commonly affected.

	Cancer distribution (%)
Peripheral zone (65% of normal gland)	80
Central zone (25% of normal gland)	5
Transitional zone (two bilateral symmetrical lobules on either side of the prostatic urethra – 10% of normal gland)	15

Pathology and prognosis

- Prostate cancers are typically adenocarcinomas.
- There is considerable uncertainty about the natural history of prostate cancer.
  - Autopsy studies reveal that 30% of men over 50 who had no symptoms of prostate cancer while alive, had histological evidence of prostate cancer at the time of death. Clearly, such indolent tumours had no effect on their survival.
  - Some contend that under the umbrella term 'prostate cancer' there is a spectrum of tumours with different growth rates. Others suggest that prostate cancer is a single disease with a very long natural history.[1]
  - It has been suggested that familial prostate cancer is a different and more aggressive form of the disease.
- Histological grade, as determined by the Gleason score, is the best predictor of tumour progression:

Gleason score	Percentage that metastasise per year
2–4 (low grade)	2
5–7 (medium grade)	5
8–10 (high grade)	13

- The staging is based on the TNM classification. Untreated localised carcinoma of the prostate results in a 5-year survival of 80%. Patients presenting with metastatic disease have a median survival of 18–24 months.

Treatment overview

- The choice of treatment depends on tumour stage and grade as well as the fitness of the patient.

Localised prostate cancer (confined to prostate capsule; T1–T2)

- Watchful waiting (no definitive treatment until signs of progression).
- Radical radiotherapy.
- Radical (total) prostatectomy.

Unfortunately, the effectiveness of these three methods of management is still not known.

Advanced prostate cancer

- Here the aims of treatment are to slow the progression of the disease and to provide symptomatic relief.
- Androgen-deprivation therapy, e.g. orchidectomy, luteinizing hormone releasing hormone (LHRH) analogues, steroidal or non-steroidal anti-androgens, oestrogens.
- Radiotherapy and palliative care.
- For primary-care practitioners it is important to be aware that starting androgen-deprivation therapy as soon as advanced disease is diagnosed (rather than reserving it until there is evidence of bone metastasis) delays progression of prostate cancer.

Prostate cancer screening

- Three methods of screening have been suggested: digital rectal examination (DRE), determination of the serum prostate-specific antigen (PSA) value, and transrectal ultrasonography (TRUS). A recent systematic review examining all the evidence related to prostate cancer screening in asymptomatic men came to the following conclusions:
  - routine testing of men to detect prostate cancer should be discouraged, irrespective of family history
  - evidence from randomised controlled trials of prostate cancer screening using PSA (or the other screening modalities) and treatment is needed before consideration should be given to funding prostate screening.[2]

Prostate screening with prostate-specific antigen: overview

The disease	Response	Comment
Is it an important problem?	Yes	See p. 63
Is the natural history well understood? (In order to determine screening interval)	No	See p. 64
Is there a recognised latent or early stage?	Possible	See p. 64

The test – PSA testing	Response	Comment
Is it simple to perform?	Yes	Blood test
Is it expensive?	No	
Is it sufficiently accurate?	No	PSA testing has a high false positive rate, see p. 68
Is it acceptable with adequate compliance?	Unsure	There is a high probability of further invasive evaluation as a result of the test. This makes the process more stressful and less acceptable to patients
Are there adequate facilities for the diagnosis and treatment of any abnormalities detected?	No	Relies on standard existing urological services

The treatment	Response
Is there an effective treatment?	Treatments remain under evaluation. Aggressive therapy is necessary in order to realise any benefit from discovering the tumour (such treatments have appreciable side-effects, morbidity, and mortality)
Does treatment at an earlier stage result in more benefit than treatment started at a later stage?	Ongoing RCTs seek to address this question. No RCTs have yet been completed

Symptoms in primary care

Prostate cancer is a slowly developing malignancy in most patients.

Urological

- Although symptoms of locally confined prostate cancer are relatively rare, because most tumours develop in the periphery of the gland, some do give rise to urological symptoms. These may be very similar to those of benign prostatic hyperplasia (BPH), which is at least four times more common, i.e.
  - obstructive symptoms: hesitancy, poor urinary flow, intermittent flow, postmicturition dribbling, and incomplete emptying
  - secondary bladder instability: urinary frequency, nocturia, and urgency.
- There is evidence that symptoms of 'prostatism' are under-reported in general practice. Specific enquiry may need to be made about such symptoms in men.[3] Three good questions are:
  - Do you get up at night to pass urine more than occasionally?
  - Is your urine flow slow?
  - Are you bothered by your bladder function?

Metastatic disease

- Bone pain.
- Back pain (*see* Chapter 18).
- Spinal cord compression.

Signs: the examination

- There are few clinical signs in early prostate cancer.
- Some advocate abdominal examination in order to detect an enlarged bladder or inguinal lymph nodes.
- Digital rectal examination (DRE) remains an important 'first line' assessment and will often detect an early lesion. Approximately 50–95% of localised prostatic tumours are palpable by DRE.
  - There is a good correlation between the observations of urologists and general practitioners when the prostate is assessed in a systematic manner[4] (*see* p. 33).
  - The consistency of the normal prostate is firm and elastic (said to be

like the tip of your nose). The following features on rectal examination are suggestive of prostate cancer:

(i) hard nodules on the smooth surface of the gland

(ii) enlarged, hard, and 'craggy' feel to the whole gland (the normal midline sulcus of the prostate becomes obliterated as the gland enlarges).

- Sensitivity of DRE ranges from 44% to 97%.
- Specificity of DRE ranges from 22% to 96%.
- The positive predictive value of DRE varies widely, from 13% to 69%. However, it is important to appreciate that the predictive value is higher under the age of 65 (25%) than over the age of 65 (12.5%). This relates to the parallel increase in the incidence of non–malignant prostate masses at the older ages.

• The predictive value of DRE may be enhanced by combination with PSA or TRUS.

Investigations

Prostate-specific antigen

• A protease produced by the prostatic epithelium.
• Levels can be raised in prostatic cancer, BPH, diagnostic examinations, and prostatitis (e.g. after biopsy).
• PSA is only a guide to prostate cancer. High values can be obtained in large, benign prostates and low values in anaplastic prostate cancer
  - PSA sensitivity, 57–99% (typically 70%)
  - PSA specificity, 59–97%.
• The cut-off point for PSA is typically 4 ng/ml. Lowering the cut-off point would increase the sensitivity (more patients detected) but reduce the specificity (more false positives).

Cut-off point	Sensitivity	Specificity
4 ng/ml	99%	87%
8 ng/ml	94%	97%

• PSA concentration varies with age, but the PSA reference range (0–4 ng/ml) does not take this into account. Suggested modifications to the reference ranges (taking age into account) are:
  - up to age 50, < 4 ng/ml
  - 60–70 years, < 7 ng/ml.

- If PSA values are increasing, referral is indicated, especially if the increase is greater than 0.8 ng/ml/year.

Serum acid phosphatase

- The prostatic component of serum acid phosphatase can be elevated in both prostatic adenocarcinoma and benign prostatic disease.
- The sensitivity for early prostate cancer is 30% (specificity 84–97%).
- If the blood test is performed after rectal examinations, false high levels may be found.

Transrectal ultrasound

- This is a method for visualising the whole gland and to guide needle biopsy.
- The relative lack of reliable information on sensitivity and specificity for TRUS alone, coupled with the expense of the procedure, continues to present problems.
- According to Brawer, the diagnostic evaluation of prostate carcinoma in primary care will continue to rely on patient symptoms and abnormal DRE and PSA results.[5]

Other investigations

- In patients with 'prostatic' symptoms it is sensible to undertake urine analysis and urea and electrolyte estimation.
- An alkaline phosphatase level may be helpful in the assessment of metastatic disease.

Local referral patterns and follow-up arrangements

- Patients with symptoms or signs suggestive of prostate cancer should be referred to an appropriate urological surgeon. Please check on the arrangements operating in your area.
- Localised prostate cancers should be followed up by annual rectal examination and 6-monthly PSA measurements. It may be possible for this review to take place in primary-care settings. (Note: although PSA values may be used to predict which men are likely to have skeletal

and nodal metastases, it is important to appreciate that, as with any investigation, there may be false negatives.)

- Patients with advanced disease need to remain under the care of an appropriate oncologist/urologist. In many areas primary-care staff are taking an active role in administering and supervising the recommended treatments.

General sources of information

British Association of Urological Surgeons (1996) *Guidelines for the Investigation and Treatment of Urological Cancers in the United Kingdom*. BAUS, London.

Chamberlain J, Melia J, Moss S, and Brown J (1997) The diagnosis, management, treatment and costs of prostate cancer in England and Wales. *Hlth Technol. Assess.* **1**(3): 1–53.

Selley S, Donovan J, Faulkner A *et al.* (1997) Diagnosis, management and screening of early localised prostate cancer. *Hlth Technol. Assess.* **1**(2): 1–96.

Stern S, Altkorn D, and Levinson W (1998) Detection of prostate and colon cancer. *JAMA* **280**: 117–18.

References

1 McNeal JE, Bostwick DG, Kindrachuk RA *et al.* (1986) Patterns of progression in prostate cancer. *Lancet* **I**: 60–3.

2 NHS Centre for Reviews and Dissemination, University of York (1997) *Effectiveness Matters – Screening for Prostate Cancer*. University of York, York.

3 Wille-Gussenhoven MJE, de Bock GH, de Beer-Buijs JM *et al.* (1997) Prostate symptoms in general practice: seriousness and inconvenience. *Scand. J. Prim. Hlth Care* **15**: 39–42.

4 Varenhorst E, Berglund K, Lofman O, and Pedersen K (1993) Inter-observer variation in assessment of the prostate by digital rectal examination. *Br. J. Urol.* **72**: 173–6.

5 Brawer MK (1993) The diagnosis of prostatic carcinoma. *Cancer* **71**: 899–905.

8

Bladder and kidney cancer

Background

Epidemiology

- Bladder cancer developed in just over 13 000 individuals in the UK during 1995.
- Bladder cancer is three times as common in men.
- Age distribution: malignant tumours of the bladder generally affect men beyond their sixth decade.
- Kidney cancer developed in 5250 individuals in 1995, being slightly more common in males.

Identifiable risk factors

- Smoking is estimated to account for half of the cases of bladder cancer in men and a quarter in women. It also increases the risk of renal cell carcinoma.
- Industrial carcinogens (up to 10% of cases). Most are associated with exposure to aromatic amines but, for some, the precise carcinogen is unclear. It is important to appreciate that latent periods of up to 40 years from the first industrial exposure can be expected. Typical occupations at risk are:
  - manufacture of rubber and rubber products
  - cable manufacturing industry
  - manufacture of dyestuffs

- manufacture of organic chemicals
- gasworks and coke ovens (in steelworks)
- rodent extermination
- sewage works
- manufacture of fire lighters and patent fuels
- laboratory work.

- Chronic irritation in some bladder cancers (diverticuli, calculi, schistoso-miasis).
- There is a familial pattern in some renal tumours. Associations of bladder cancer with genetic polymorphisms of glutathione S-transferase and N-acetyl transferase have been demonstrated.

Pathology and prognosis

- In the UK most bladder tumours (90%) are transitional cell carcinomas, commonly located in the base and lateral walls of the bladder. The tumours can be papillary or solid, multiple or solitary.
- Worldwide, the most common cause of bladder cancer is schistoso-miasis, which results in squamous carcinoma.
- Superficial bladder tumours (T1) account for 80% of bladder cancers. Very few progress to muscle invasion and the risk of metastatic disease is small (10-year survival is 70%).
- Muscle-invasive bladder cancer (T3) is a life-threatening condition with a 10-year survival of less than 20%.
- Renal-cell carcinomas are adenocarcinomas.
- The prognosis for tumours confined to the kidney is reasonable, with a 5-year survival of 50% after radical nephrectomy.

Treatment overview

- Treatment options for bladder cancer consist of transurethral resection followed by regular cystoscopic surveillance, immunotherapy (e.g. intravesical bacille Calmette–Guérin (BCG)), and intravesical chemotherapy (e.g. metomycin or epirubicin). More advanced tumours may require cystectomy and/or radiotherapy.
- Radical or partial nephrectomy is the treatment of choice for uncompli-cated renal tumours. This may be supplemented by hormone treatment with progestogens, or biological therapy with interferon and inter-leukin–2. It is generally agreed that chemotherapy is ineffective for renal-cell carcinoma.

Screening for bladder and kidney cancer

- A recent systematic review does not recommend the use of routine urinalysis for microscopic haematuria as a screening test. It is neither sufficiently sensitive nor specific and has a poor predictive value for urological malignancies.[1]

Symptoms in primary care

Macroscopic haematuria[2,3]

- Amongst referred populations, macroscopic haematuria is highly sensitive for bladder cancers (83%) and urethral cancer (66%). The sensitivity of haematuria for renal cancer was 48% and for any urological cancer 22%.
- The positive predictive value of macroscopic haematuria is higher (41%) in patients aged over 40.
- In a series of 212 consecutive patients with bladder tumours from Scandinavia, the presenting symptom was macroscopic haematuria in 79% of patients. Unfortunately, women with haematuria suffered a longer delay in the diagnosis of their bladder tumour.

Microscopic haematuria

- Defined as a positive result on dipstix testing and/or greater than five red blood cells per high-power field (HPF) or around 12 500 red blood cells/ml.
- Approximately 10% of healthy, and presumably asymptomatic, adults have one or more red blood cells (RBCs) per HPF.
- As can be seen from the table below, microscopic haematuria is common in asymptomatic adults.

Unselected community studies of microscopic haematuria in men

	Messing et al.[4]	Britton et al.[5]
Total number screened	1340	2356
Age	>50 years	>60 years
Number with haematuria	283 (21%)	474 (20%)
Number undergoing further evaluation	192	319
Number with asymptomatic urological cancers	16	17

- In studies of selected referred patients, 2–11% were reported as having urothelial malignancies.
- In evaluating patients with asymptomatic microscopic haematuria, it has been suggested that other risk factors (such as age >40 and persistence of haematuria) should play a greater role in the decision regarding further investigations.[6,7] Unfortunately, the research evidence to support this view is absent and hence the guideline from the Scottish Intercollegiate Guidelines Network (SIGN) recommends continued investigation of all cases of asymptomatic haematuria (but *see* p. 76).
- It is important to appreciate that in one series less than 10% of patients with bladder tumours had haematuria.[1] Moreover, excretion of red blood cells in the urine of patients with urothelial malignancies may be intermittent.[4] In view of this, Connelly has suggested that evaluation of microscopic haematuria in patients over the age of 50 should be based on its initial discovery.[8]

Non-specific urinary symptoms

For example, frequency, urgency, dysuria, loin pain, pelvic pain, and bladder outflow obstruction.
- In a study in Scandinavia, 20% of patients with bladder cancer had cystitis-like symptoms.[2] These patients represent the group with the longest delay in diagnosis.
- For renal-cell carcinomas flank pain is the second most common symptom after haematuria, occurring in 40% of patients.

Kidney tumours

- In addition to haematuria and flank pain, renal-cell carcinomas may first present with symptoms of metastases, e.g. to bone (pain) or lung (cough/haemoptysis).
- One-third of patients may complain of weight loss (*see* Chapter 18).
- In some series, 25–30% of such patients have no symptoms related specifically to the kidney, and tumours are found incidentally by radiological or ultrasound examination.

Signs: the examination

- Examination by the general practitioner is usually quite unremarkable.
- In the presence of non-specific urinary symptoms, the kidneys and

bladder should be assessed for enlargement and tenderness and a digital rectal examination should be performed in males. One-quarter of patients with renal-cell carcinoma present with a palpable mass.
- In 10–20% of patients with renal-cell carcinoma there may be an associated fever, hypertension, or anaemia.

Investigations

- Any investigations (either radiological or laboratory based) should only be undertaken if the practitioner considers that the outcome of that investigation will materially affect his or her decision. As with any investigation there may be false negatives.
- All patients with macroscopic haematuria need referral.
- All patients with microscopic haematuria require investigation (Figure 8.1) and possible referral (*see* p. 76).

Figure 8.1 Investigation of patients with microscopic haematuria.

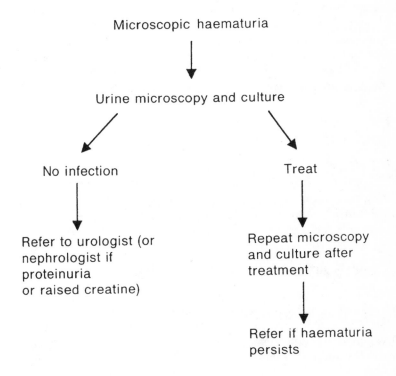

Practical considerations

- Most dipstix detect about eight red blood cells per high-power field.
- False-positive reactions on dipstix may be caused by bacterial peroxidases, or antiseptic solutions.
- False-negative reactions on dipstix may be caused by acidic urine, excess ascorbic acid, or rifampicin.
- To assess haematuria, mid-stream urine (MSU) samples need to be fresh, reaching the laboratory within 2 hours of being produced.
- Urine cytology: although this may be useful for follow-up, its sensitivity for diagnosis is quite low, at 55%.
- Renal-cell carcinoma may be associated with a variety of abnormal findings, e.g. elevated ESR (55% of cases), anaemia (33% of cases), abnormal liver function tests (15% of cases), hypercalcaemia (5% of cases), and polycythemia (3% of cases).

Follow-up and detection of recurrence

- Cystoscopic suveillance is essential in superficial (T1) bladder tumours, as recurrence will occur in about 50% of cases. After a period of 3 years without recurrence, outpatient surveillance with cytology and/or ultrasound may be recommended.
- Bladder tumours are associated with a risk of developing further urothelial tumours, e.g. bladder, ureters, and renal pelvises.
- The follow-up of renal-cell carcinomas must involve an appropriate specialist team. Following radical nephrectomy, most recurrences are diagnosed by a careful history and chest radiography.

Local referral patterns

- Many areas now have open-access haematuria clinics for direct referral of patients. Please refer to your local referral guidelines for such clinics.

General sources of information

British Association of Urological Surgeons (1996) *Guidelines for the Investigation and Treatment of Urological Cancers in the United Kingdom*. BAUS, London.
Cancer Research Campaign (1997) *Bladder Cancer – UK*. Cancer Research Campaign, London.
Scottish Intercollegiate Guidelines Network (SIGN) (1997) *Investigation of Asympto-*

matic Microscopic Haematuria in Adults. SIGN publication No. 17. SIGN, Edinburgh.

References

1   Froom P, Froom J, and Ribak J (1997) Asymptomatic microscopic haematuria – is investigation necessary? *J. Clin. Epidemiol.* **50**: 1197–200.

2   Mommsen S, Aagaard J, and Sell A (1983) Presenting symptoms, treatment delay and survival in bladder cancer. *Scand. J. Urol. Nephrol.* **17**: 163–7.

3   Buntix F and Wanters H (1997) The diagnostic value of macroscopic haematuria in diagnosing urological cancers; a meta analysis. *Fam. Pract.* **14**: 63–8.

4   Messing EM, Young TB, Hunt VB *et al.* (1992) Home screening for haematuria; results of a multi-clinic study. *J. Urol.* **148**: 289–92.

5   Britton JP, Dowell AC, Whelan P, and Harris CM (1992) A community study of bladder cancer screening by the detection of occult urinary bleeding. *J. Urol.* **148**: 788–90.

6   Froom B, Ribak J, and Benbassat J (1984) Significance of microhaematuria in young adults. *BMJ* **288**: 20–2.

7   Mohr DN, Offord KP, Owen RA, and Melton J (1986) Asymptomatic micro-haematuria and urologic disease: a population based study. *JAMA* **256**: 224–9.

8   Connelly J (1991) Microscopic haematuria. In: RJ Panzer, ER Black, and P Griner (eds) *Diagnostic Strategies for Common Medical Problems.* ACP, Philadelphia.

9

Testicular cancer

Background

Epidemiology

- Testicular tumours are most common in young men aged 18–45.
- In the UK there were 1380 new cases in 1995.
- Accounts for 1% of male cancers.
- Four and a half times more common in Caucasian males.
- Most common cancer in men aged 20–34.

Identifiable risk factors

- Developmental abnormality, i.e. testicular maldescent (cryptorchidism) (risk also applies to contralateral testis). Such individuals have 2.5–4.0 times the risk of the general population (10% of patients).
- Previous cancer in opposite testis (4% risk of second cancer).
- Family history of testicular cancer, testicular maldescent, or cryptorchidism. It has been estimated that the relative risk for first-degree relatives of a patient is increased by a factor of 3–10 (at least 2% of patients are in this category).
- Previous inguinal/testicular problems in childhood – mumps orchitis, inguinal hernia, testicular torsion, hydrocele.
- Other developmental abnormalities – gonadal dysgenesis, Klinefelter's syndrome.

Pathology and prognosis

- Most testicular cancers (95%) are germ-cell tumours – 40% of these are seminomas, 60% non-seminomas (mainly teratomas but also embryonal carcinoma, choriocarcinoma, and yolk-cell carcinoma).
- Four per cent of testicular cancers are lymphomas (mainly found in men over the age of 50).
- Teratomas can grow very rapidly, seminomas grow more slowly.
- Staging is performed by clinical examination, CT scanning of the chest and abdomen together with estimation of tumour markers.
- Ninety per cent of seminomas have a 5-year survival of 86%. Detection of any human chorionic gonadotrophin (HCG) or serum lactate dehydrogenase (LDH) lowers this to 72% (in 10% of cases).
- The prognosis of teratoma can be divided into three categories based on marker levels:[1]

Proportion of non-seminomas (all with no non-pulmonary visceral metastasis)	α-Fetoprotein	Human chorionic gonadotrophin	Lactate dehydrogenase	Five-year survival
56%	<1000 mg/ml	<5000 IU/l	<1.5 × upper limit normal	92%
28%	1000–10 000 mg/ml	5000–15 000 IU/l	1.5–10 × upper limit normal	80%
16%	>10 000 mg/ml	or >50 000 IU/l	or >10 × upper limit normal	48%

- General practitioners have an important role in encouraging early diagnosis and referral. A poorer prognosis is seen with advanced disease and there is a clear correlation between the interval from onset of symptoms to diagnosis and the stage of the disease, i.e. delay in diagnosis is associated with poorer outcomes.

Treatment overview

- Testicular cancer is broadly divided into seminoma and non-seminoma for treatment planning because seminomas are more sensitive to radiotherapy.

- Surgery is the initial treatment for all testicular tumours (inguinal orchidectomy).
- Seminoma is highly sensitive to both radiotherapy and chemotherapy. Nearly all relapses occur in the para-aortic lymph nodes and the standard treatment for stage I seminoma is radiotherapy to this area. Relapse is most common in the first 12–18 months.
- Orchidectomy and surveillance for low-risk stage I teratomas are usually recommended, e.g. tumour marker measurement monthly for 1 year and 2-monthly for a second year, with regular clinical examinations, chest radiography, and CT scanning.
- Orchidectomy and chemotherapy are usually indicated for high-risk stage I teratomas.
- Patients with more extensive metastatic teratomas require combination chemotherapy according to nationally agreed trials. Such patients should be managed at a cancer centre.

Screening for testicular cancer

- Although screening by routine testicular self-examination has been proposed, no rigorous studies have been conducted to assess its benefit. There is certainly no evidence that practising regular self-examination influences delay in diagnosis.[2]
- Primary-care staff can best work to raise the public awareness of testicular cancer amongst young men. This should also include information on the curability of the condition.

Symptoms in primary care

Early symptoms

- Most common symptom (over 86% of patients):
  - painless mass in testicle (i.e. enlarged testicle or a lump in the testicle).
- Other symptoms:
  - testicular discomfort or pain (31% of patients); a dragging sensation has been reported in 29% of patients
  - newly acquired hydrocele in young males
  - 'epididymitis' that fails to settle completely or epididymo-orchitis not responding to antibiotics, or recurrent 'epididymo-orchitis' (15% of patients)
  - a recent history of trauma may be present in up to 10% of patients.

Later symptoms

- Metastatic, e.g. back pain (5%), dyspnoea (pleural effusion), abdominal discomfort or swelling (para-aortic lymph nodes), haemoptysis.
- Gynaecomastia may occur in up to 10% of patients with elevated HCG levels.

Signs: the examination

- Careful clinical examination of the testes still remains the best method of detecting a tumour. An attempt needs to be made to distinguish between lumps arising from the body of the testis and other intrascrotal swellings.
- Abnormal firmness or hard swelling in the body of the testes is the most reliable finding. Unusual differences between one testicle and the other may also be helpful.
- It is important to have a high index of suspicion in cases of testicular pain and tenderness. The most common error is to mistake a tumour for epididymitis because the swollen testis is tender. In one study, 55% of patients eventually found to have cancer were treated initially for epididymitis.[3]
- Since, in some cases, metastatic disease may give the first symptoms and cure may still be possible, palpation of the testes should be performed when there are unexplained symptoms (e.g. abdominal, chest, or neck and back pain) in younger males.

Investigations

- Urine for microscopy, culture and sensitivity in cases of 'epididymitis'. Absence of pyuria indicates a need for further investigation.
- The initial evaluation of a testicular mass is by ultrasonography. Tumour markers and testicular ultrasound requests are often best arranged by the urologist after referral if he or she considers it appropriate (it is important to check on the local arrangements operating in your area).
- Tumour markers (e.g. α-fetoprotein (AFP), β-HCG) can detect early or small-volume disease, but are most useful for early determination of relapse in previously treated teratoma patients.
- Markers are seldom useful in seminomas as only a small proportion have elevated β-HCG. Any elevation of AFP in seminomas indicates unidentified teratoma.

- LDH is a non-specific marker but correlates with the volume of metastatic disease and is used as a prognostic factor (*see* p. 80).
- Following referral, additional staging investigations may be performed (e.g. chest radiography, CT scan of abdomen and pelvis). Biopsy of the contralateral testis may be advised, especially with a history of maldescent, atrophy, or infertility.

Follow-up and detection of recurrence

- Follow-up is an integral part of management (*see* p. 81) and the majority of such follow-up will take place under specialist supervision.
- In general, the surveillance should be greater but over a shorter time period for non-seminomas compared to seminomas.
- Since the majority of patients with testicular cancer who receive chemotherapy are curable, it is important to be aware of possible long-term effects of platinum-based treatments.
    - effects on fertility (where appropriate sperm storage should be offered to men who may require chemotherapy or radiotherapy)
    - secondary leukaemias.

Local referral patterns

- Any patients suspected of having a testicular malignancy should be seen rapidly (within 1–2 weeks) by an appropriate specialist.
- It is important to check on your local referral patterns for the diagnosis and management of testicular malignancies.

General sources of information

British Association of Urological Surgeons (1996) *Guidelines for the Investigation and Treatment of Urological Cancers in the United Kingdom.* BAUS, London.
Cancer Research Campaign (1998) *Testicular Cancer – UK.* Cancer Research Campaign, London.
Scottish Intercollegiate Guidelines Network (SIGN) (1998) *Management of Adult Testicular Germ Cell Tumours.* (SIGN publication No. 28). SIGN, Edinburgh.

References

1   International Germ Cell Cancer Collaborative Group (1997) International germ cell consensus classification: a prognostic factor-based staging system for metastatic germ cell cancers. *J. Clin. Oncol.* **15**: 594–603.

2 Buetow SA (1996) Testicular cancer: to screen or not to screen? *J. Med. Screen.* **3**: 3–6.

3 Vogt HB and McHale MS (1992) Testicular cancer. Role of primary care physicians in screening and education. *Postgrad. Med.* **92**: 93–101.

10

Ovarian cancer

Background

Epidemiology

- Ovarian cancer is the most common gynaecological cancer in women.
- In 1995, just under 6000 women were diagnosed with the disease and it resulted in over 4000 deaths.
- Most cancers (90%) occur in women over the age of 45 years (majority postmenopausal, with the peak at age 65–75).

Identifiable risk factors

- Ovulation: the risk of ovarian cancer **decreases** with increasing parity, anovulation, and oral contraceptive use (relative risk of oral contraceptive use versus no contraceptive = 0.66, relative risk of any term pregnancy versus nulliparity = 0.47).
- Family history:
  - This is present in about 7% of women with ovarian cancer. A family history of ovarian cancer in a first- or second-degree relative is one of the strongest risk factors for epithelial ovarian cancer.

	Relative risk
One first- or second-degree relative with ovarian cancer	3.1
Two or three relatives with ovarian cancer	4.6

- In half of the families with such a history, there may be a dominantly inherited gene. Three distinct hereditary syndromes have been identified in ovarian cancer families:
  (i) site-specific ovarian cancer
  (ii) breast cancer–ovarian cancer syndrome
  (iii) cancer family syndromes (Lynch type II, i.e. family clustering of tumours including colorectal, endometrial, ovary and breast cancer).
- The tumour-suppressor genes BRCA-1/BRCA-2 have been suggested as markers for some of the familial cancer syndromes. Women with mutations to the BRCA-1/BRCA-2 genes are at increased risk for the development of breast and ovarian cancer. The estimated lifetime risk of ovarian cancer in women with BRCA-1 mutations is 45%, and in women with BRCA-2 mutations, 25% (see Chapter 3). Recently, it has been suggested that the regular use of oral contraceptives may reduce the chance of developing ovarian cancer among women who inherit BRCA-1 or BRCA-2.

Pathology and prognosis

- Ovarian cancer is not a single disease but represents a group of cancers arising from a variety of different cell types.
- Histological classification is complex but the majority (90%) are of epithelial origin.
- Non-epithelial ovarian cancer includes germ-cell tumours and sex-cord stromal tumours. Germ-cell tumours account for 1–2% of ovarian tumours, are most common in young women (aged 15–19) and have a better prognosis than epithelial ovarian cancers.
- The tumour spreads from the ovaries locally and also by peritoneal seeding.

Prognosis by stage

Stage		Five-year relative survival (%)
I	Cancer limited to ovaries	78
II	Cancer limited to pelvis	59
III	Cancer extending to abdominal cavity	23
IV	Metastases to distant sites	14

- Although patients with local disease confined to the ovaries have a favourable prognosis, more than half of patients with ovarian cancer present at stage III or IV.

Treatment overview

The usual treatment for stage I low-grade disease is surgery alone (bilateral oophorectomy and omentectomy), while more advanced disease may be treated with surgery followed by adjuvant chemotherapy (based on the best available trial evidence).

Ovarian cancer screening

- In view of the insidious nature of epithelial ovarian cancer, with no specific symptoms in the early stages (*see* p. 88), it has been suggested that screening should be considered.
- Unfortunately, the natural history of ovarian cancer is not well understood and there isn't a recognised latent or early stage.
- Three tests have been advocated for early detection of ovarian cancer: bimanual rectovaginal pelvic examination, cancer antigen 125 (CA-125) tumour marker in the serum, and/or ultrasonography imaging techniques.
- Physical examination has proved too insensitive and non-specific to be used as a screening test – it has been estimated that only one case of early-stage ovarian cancer can be detected in 10 000 routine pelvic examinations.
- Eighty per cent of epithelial ovarian cancers produce CA-125. A positive screening result is defined as a serum level greater than 35 microunits per millilitre. Unfortunately only about 50% of patients with stage I disease have elevated CA-125 levels (risk of false negatives). CA-125 levels may also be raised in certain benign conditions such as fibroids, endometriosis, and early pregnancy.
- CA-125 with abdominal ultrasound has positive predictive value of 26.8%, specificity of 99.9%, and sensitivity of 58%. Thus in accordance with the rule of SpPin (*see* Appendix 1: 'if a test has sufficiently high specificity, a positive result rules in the disorder'), CA-125 and abdominal ultrasound may be useful in supporting the diagnosis of ovarian cancer. However, in view of the lower sensitivity, a negative result cannot be used to rule out ovarian cancer.
- Screening studies using transvaginal ultrasonography have demonstrated a higher specificity of screening than studies using transabdominal ultrasonography. Concomitant colour Doppler imaging reduces the number of false positives (sensitivity 100%, with false positives of 0.9%).
- According to a recent systematic review, although three large RCTs are in progress (*see* below), no RCTs of screening for ovarian cancer have

been completed. Bell *et al.* (1998) concluded that in the absence of evidence of effectiveness, it would be premature to establish any kind of screening programme.

The ongoing RCTs for ovarian cancer screening

Study	Protocol	Expected date of completion
Barts (UK)	CA-125 test followed by ultrasound in those testing positive	2003
ERTOCS (UK/Europe)	Transvaginal ultrasound	2005
NIHPLCO (USA)	Transvaginal ultrasound plus CA-125 plus pelvic examination	2005

- As the overall incidence of ovarian cancer in the general female population is low, screening has also been advocated in the high-risk population of women with a family history of ovarian cancer. A further study has just commenced examining annual transvaginal ultrasound and CA-125 estimation in this group.

Symptoms in primary care

- In early-stage ovarian cancer there may be minimal or no symptoms, and symptoms are often non-specific even in the more advanced stages. It is therefore extremely important to be aware of a patient's cancer family history for assessing the risk for ovarian cancer.
- Abdominal discomfort or pain (e.g. resulting from torsion or traction) are the most common presenting complaints.
- A slightly smaller proportion of women first complain of a sensation of distension or feeling a lump.
- As the tumour enlarges, patients may complain of a sense of pelvic weight or pressure. Symptoms may also arise from compression effects of the tumour within the abdomen, e.g. dyspepsia, constipation, urinary frequency, ankle oedema.
- In a woman with persistent, otherwise unexplained gastrointestinal symptoms (e.g. abdominal distension, discomfort or pain, dyspepsia, weight loss, and bowel dysfunction) ovarian cancer should be excluded.
- In 15% of patients there is postmenopausal bleeding or, in younger women, menstrual irregularity.

Signs: the examination

- The most important positive sign of ovarian cancer is a pelvic mass on vaginal examination, particularly one that is irregular and fixed. Unfortunately, bimanual pelvic examination has low specificity and low sensitivity and should not be relied on to exclude ovarian enlargement. There is evidence that the false-positive rate is high when examinations are performed by a gynaecologist (but even higher when performed by GPs and practice nurses).
- Any hard abdominal mass arising from the pelvis is highly suggestive of ovarian cancer, especially in the presence of ascites.
- The ovaries in a postmenopausal woman should not be palpable. If either ovary can be felt, malignancy should be excluded.

Investigations and local referral patterns

- If a patient has symptoms or signs suggestive of ovarian malignancy, then an urgent referral should be made to a gynaecologist with a specialist interest in ovarian cancer.
- A pelvic ultrasound (if available through open access) may provide additional evidence favouring referral but should **not** be used to prevent a clinical referral decision. **Vaginal ultrasonography** is more accurate than transabdominal ultrasound.
- None of the tumour markers currently available are sufficiently sensitive or specific to detect ovarian cancer at an early stage (*see* p. 87).
- Ovarian cysts are present in 6% of asymptomatic postmenopausal women. Decisions on treatment are often based on age, menopausal status, the size of the cysts, and whether the structure is unilocular or multilocular. It is important to refer to your local cancer centre management guidelines but, in general, persistent ovarian cysts or tumours in patients over the age of 40 should be investigated further to establish their benign status.

Follow-up and detection of recurrence

- Patients are followed up at the discretion of the gynaecological oncologists.
- CA-125 has an established role in monitoring the disease during treatment, for surveillance during follow-up (often for over 5 years), and the trend of CA-125 can give prognostic information.

General sources of information

Bell R, Petticrew M, Luengo S, and Sheldon TA (1998) Screening for ovarian cancer: a systematic review. *Hlth Technol. Assess.* **2**(2): 1–84.

Cancer Research Campaign (1997) *Ovarian Cancer – UK*. Cancer Research Campaign, London.

11

Endometrial cancer

Background

Epidemiology

- In the UK there were just over 4000 new cases of endometrial cancer in 1995.
- It is essentially a disease of postmenopausal women (median age 61 years), with at least three-quarters of cases occurring after the menopause. However, 20% of cases will be diagnosed before the menopause and 5% below the age of 40 years.

Identifiable risk factors

- Obesity: women 21–50 lb (10–23 kg) overweight have three times the risk of developing endometrial cancer; and for those more than 50 lb (23 kg) overweight the risk is increased tenfold.
- Low parity (the risk is doubled for nulliparous women compared to women with one child).
- Prolonged oestrogen stimulation (endogenous or exogenous). Women with oestrogen-secreting tumours or polycystic ovary syndrome are at increased risk. The use of exogenous oestrogen unopposed by progesterone increases the risk of endometrial cancer by over fivefold. In contrast, the use of the combined oral contraceptive pill acts as a protective factor.
- Menstrual history: late menopause after age 52 increases the risk 2.4 times. Menarche after the age of 15 years acts as a protective factor.

- Tamoxifen therapy has been shown to result in a slight risk for endometrial cancer (*see* Chapter 6).
- Diabetes and hypertension: the evidence in favour of these as independent risk factors is controversial.
- Genetic factors: positive family histories are present in approximately 15% of cases. Endometrial adenocarcinoma can occur as one component of the Lynch type II family cancer syndrome (*see* p. 86).

Pathology and prognosis

- Most endometrial cancers (80%) are adenocarcinomas. Others are papillary serous, mucinous, clear-cell, squamous-cell, and mixed.
- Endometrial adenocarcinoma has a good prognosis if the condition is identified early.

Stage		Five-year survival (%)
I	Confined to endometrium (70–80% of patients)	70
II	Invasion of cervix	50
III	Spread to pelvic tissues	25
IV	Spread to bladder/rectum/distant sites	5

- Endometrial hyperplasia with atypia is a premalignant condition.

Treatment overview

- Most women are treated surgically with hysterectomy and bilateral salpingo-oophorectomy.
- Where the disease is known to involve the endocervix, consideration will be given to performing a Wertheim's hysterectomy.
- Postoperative pelvic irradiation will be offered to certain groups of patients, e.g. those with more than 50% invasion of the myometrium, where there is involvement of the endocervix, and in patients with bulky or poorly differentiated tumours.

Screening for endometrial cancer

- There is currently no evidence in favour of screening for endometrial cancer.

- It has been suggested that control of body weight may have an effect on reducing the risk of endometrial cancer.

Symptoms in primary care

- The cardinal symptom for endometrial cancer is inappropriate vaginal bleeding (occasionally preceded by brownish, watery discharge, which may be offensive).
- Because of the age distribution of the disease, the prime symptom is postmenopausal bleeding (defined as bleeding that occurs after 1 year of amenorrhoea in women not receiving hormone replacement therapy). According to Good, postmenopausal women should undergo endometrial assessment in the following circumstances:[1]
  - when bleeding occurs in the absence of hormone replacement therapy
  - when bleeding occurs after a 1-year regimen of continuous–combined hormone replacement therapy
  - when bleeding occurs at an unexpected time during cyclic replacement therapy.

  Recently the American College of Obstetricians and Gynecologists recommended endometrial assessment in women who are taking continuous–combined HRT and have bleeding for more than 6 months after starting treatment, and for any prolonged or irregular bleeding in women taking cyclic HRT.
- In younger women (20% of cases), the presenting complaint is inter-menstrual bleeding or menorrhagia.
- Endometrial cancer may also give rise to pelvic pain but this is an infrequent presentation.

Signs: the examination

- The enlargement of the uterus occurs only when the disease is advanced and is not a reliable sign.

Investigations

- FBC should be performed if the bleeding has been persistent or heavy.
- Patients with postmenopausal bleeding should be referred to a gynaecologist in accordance with locally agreed guidelines. Following referral, a number of methods of endometrial assessment are used as

the actual prevalence of serious pathology in women with postmenopausal bleeding is estimated to be less than 5%.[2]

- Outpatient endometrial sampling (e.g. Pipelle sampler):
(i) sensitivity ranges from 88 to 97%
(ii) sampling is less sensitive with early lesions, with polyps, and when the abnormality is focal rather than global.
- Endovaginal ultrasound (EVUS): Smith-Bindman *et al.* have shown that in a population of postmenopausal women with vaginal bleeding, EVUS (using a threshold level of >5 mm as abnormal) has a sensitivity of 96% for detection of endometrial cancer.[3]
- Hysteroscopy: this allows direct visualisation and biopsy of early-localised endometrial lesions. It is the 'gold standard' against which other methods of endometrial assessment are compared.
- Dilatation and curettage (D & C):
(i) the usefulness of D & C as a diagnostic tool has been repeatedly questioned
(ii) several studies have indicated that a significant proportion of endometrial lesions are not detected by D & C.
- **A negative cervical cytology report does not exclude endometrial cancer.**

Follow-up and local referral patterns

- Agboola *et al.* concluded that intensive follow-up of women with endometrial cancer does not result in improved survival.[4]
- However, it is important to check on local arrangements for referral and follow-up of patients with endometrial cancer. Many units follow up such patients at regular intervals for a minimum of 5 years.

References

1 Good AE (1997) Diagnostic options for the assessment of postmenopausal bleeding. *Mayo Clin. Proc.* **72**: 345–9.
2 Carlson KJ (1998) Vaginal ultrasonography to evaluate postmenopausal bleeding. *JAMA* **280**: 1529–30.
3 Smith-Bindman R, Kerlikowske K, Feldstein VA *et al.* (1998) Endovaginal ultrasound to exclude endometrial cancer and other endometrial abnormalities. *JAMA* **280**: 1510–17.
4 Agboola OO, Grunfeld E, Coyle D, and Perry GA (1997) Costs and benefits of routine follow-up after curative treatment for endometrial cancer. *Can. Med. Assoc. J.* **157**: 879–86.

12

Cervical cancer

Background

Epidemiology

- There were just under 3500 new cases of invasive cervical cancer in the UK during 1995.
- In 1994, 1369 women in England and Wales died from cervical cancer.
- In England and Wales, 18 753 women were registered in 1988 as having carcinoma *in situ* (including grade III cervical intraepithelial neoplasia, CIN3).
- Although only 15% of cases occur in women under the age of 35, it is the most common cancer in this age group.
- It is more common in women of lower socio-economic status.

Identifiable risk factors

- Early first intercourse (coitus before age 17 doubles risk).
- Women with multiple sexual partners (doubles risk).
- Promiscuous male partner (more than 15 partners) (eight times risk).
- Smoking (doubles risk).
- Sexually transmitted viral infection (especially human papillomavirus type 16 infection – present in 93% of cervical cancers).
- Genetic susceptibility (a variation in the *p53* tumour-suppressor gene may increase the risk sevenfold).

Pathology and prognosis

- High-grade cervical intraepithelial neoplasia (CIN) is considered to be a premalignant condition. Screening for dysplastic cells which are associated with CIN is the basis of the cervical screening programme.
- Ninety-five per cent of cervical cancers are squamous carcinomas. The remainder are adenocarcinomas.
- Macroscopically, CIN is invisible to the naked eye; cervical cancer can appear as a proliferative growth at the cervix with surface ulceration, or a diffusely infiltrating tumour.

Prognosis and stage for cervical cancer

Stage		Five-year survival (%)
1A	Microinvasive disease limited to cervix	>95
1B	Confined to cervix with invasion >5 mm depth from surface	80
2A	Extension to upper two-thirds of vagina	60–70
2B	Extension to parametrium	50
3	Extension to lower vagina/pelvic wall	25
4	Involvement of bladder/rectum/distant sites	<10

Treatment overview

- For CIN the treatment choice lies between local destructive therapy (e.g. laser, cryosurgery) or local excision by cone biopsy.
- For invasive cervical cancer the treatment depends on the stage. Stage 1A is often managed by simple hysterectomy or large cone biopsy. Stages 1B and 2A require more radical surgery. More advanced stages are often considered for radiotherapy.

The cervical screening programme

The general practitioner and the primary healthcare team have very important roles and responsibilities in relation to this programme. Most recently these have been outlined in the booklet *Cervical Smear Results Explained: A Guide for Primary Care.*[1] In particular, **it is important**:

- To co-operate and collaborate with the local health authority in ensuring the effectiveness of the computerised call–recall system.
- To encourage **all** eligible women to have a smear. According to

Woodman *et al.* there is a widespread, but mistaken, belief that social and behavioural characteristics can be used to identify a group of high-risk women who would benefit most from intensive cytological surveillance. For this to be possible, it would be necessary to identify characteristics that are at least 50 times more common in women with cervical cancer than in those who remain disease free.[2]

- To improve the quality of the smears taken:
  - it is the responsibility of the smear taker to visualise the cervix to ensure that the whole of the transformation zone has been swiped
  - endocervical cells and/or immature metaplastic cells are indicators of transformation zone sampling; such evidence should be present in the majority of women under the age of 50
  - 5–10% of smears are inadequate or unsuitable, often due to poor technique (e.g. inadequate fixation, poor spreading)
  - according to Lo and Jordan,[3] adding a cytology brush sample to the Pap smear resulted in a significant increase in the rate of Pap smears that detected cells – the cytology brush was significantly better than the spatula for detecting endocervical cells but not significantly better for detecting metaplastic cells
  - in older women the transformation zone moves into the os. In order to reach this area a spatula with a pointed and extended tip has been recommended as there is evidence that it has a better pick up rate for dyskaryotic cells.
- To deal effectively with results and patients:

Follow-up protocol based on smear result

Evidence of neoplasia	Inflammation	Action recommended
Inadequate		Repeat in 3 months After 3 consecutive inadequates refer for colposcopy
Negative		Normal recall
Negative	Mild, moderate, or severe	Normal recall
Negative	With an infection (no nuclear changes)	Normal recall
Borderline (1st) (i.e. smears in which there is doubt as to whether or not nuclear changes reflect true dyskaryosis)	Including wart virus	Repeat in 6 months (if negative, repeat smear yearly for 2 years then to 3-yearly recall)

Borderline (2nd)	Repeat in 3 months
Borderline (3rd)	Refer for colposcopy
Mild dyskaryosis (1st)	Repeat in 3 months (if negative, repeat smear yearly for 2 years then to 3-yearly recall)
Mild dyskaryosis (2nd) (i.e. persistence after 6 months)	Refer for colposcopy
Moderate/severe dyskaryosis	Refer for colposcopy
Glandular neoplasia/ severe dyskaryosis ? invasive	Refer to gynae-oncologist

- Essentially colposcopy is indicated if there are:
  - borderline changes on two or three occasions
  - mild dyskaryosis on two occasions
  - moderate dyskaryosis on one occasion
  - severe dyskaryosis on one occasion.

Cervical cytology screening: overview

The disease	Response	Comment
Is it an important problem?	Yes	See p. 95
Is the natural history well understood? (In order to determine screening interval)	No. The progression through the CIN stages is uncertain with some regression	
Is there a recognised latent or early stage?	Yes	Dysplasia; severe dysplasia predicts CIN3

The test – cervical smear	Response	Comment
Is it simple to perform?	Reasonable	Requires adequate training. Primary-care staff vary in their ability to submit adequate smears
Is it expensive?	Reasonable	Equipment and staff
Is it sufficiently accurate?	Reasonable	In a review of 100 cervical cancer cases, 9% had

		a normal smear in the past 5 years
Is it acceptable with adequate compliance?	Reasonable	Some concerns about compliance especially amongst the groups most at risk
Are there adequate facilities for the diagnosis and treatment of any abnormalities detected?	Yes	It is important to check on local arrangements for referral and follow-up

The treatment	Response
Is there any effective treatment?	Yes
Does treatment at an earlier stage result in more benefit than treatment started at a later stage?	Yes (although no RCTs have been undertaken, population-based comparisons (e.g. Iceland versus UK) have provided supportive evidence)

Symptoms in primary care

- The premalignant phase of the disease, cervical intraepithelial neoplasia, is not associated with any symptoms or signs, hence the importance of the smear.
- Early symptoms of invasive cancer:
  - irregular bleeding – particularly postcoital bleeding, bleeding noted after micturition/defecation, or postmenopausal bleeding; this is the most common symptom in individuals with invasive cervical cancer
  - vaginal discharge – initially non-specific; later this discharge may be blood-tinged or offensive.
- Later symptoms are related to local spread, e.g. renal dysfunction (due to ureteric obstruction), haematuria, rectal bleeding, low back and sacral pain.

Signs: the examination

- In order to diagnose early invasive cancer it is important to have a high index of suspicion and a willingness to carry out a full pelvic examination for relatively minor symptoms.

- **Speculum examination:** any lesion on the cervix (e.g. nodule, small ulcer, or an inflamed cervix) that bleeds easily on gentle examination should be regarded with suspicion, even if the smear is reported as normal.
- **Cytological examination of cervical smears has detection rather than diagnostic accuracy.**[2] A negative cytology report **does not** exclude cervical cancer and can simply cause delays or provide false reassurance. If there is a suspicious lesion on the cervix, arrange urgent referral – **do not** wait for the smear report.

Follow-up of patients in primary care

After cervical biopsy and treatment for CIN	Smear after 6 months (if negative, repeat smears yearly for 5 years then repeat every 3 years)
After total hysterectomy for CIN, or if CIN is found in the hysterectomy specimen	Smear after 6 months (if negative repeat smear 1 year later, i.e. 18 months after hysterectomy). If these two smears both give negative results, then no further screening smear tests are generally required

General sources of information

Austoker J (1995) *Cancer Prevention in Primary Care.* BMJ, London.
Cancer Research Campaign (1994) *Cancer of the Cervix Uteri.* Cancer Research Campaign, London.
Cancer Research Campaign (1994) *Cervical Cancer Screening.* Cancer Research Campaign, London.
Ridsdale L (1995) *Evidence-based General Practice. A Critical Reader.* Saunders, London.

References

1   Austoker J and Davey C (1997) *Cervical smear results explained: a guide for primary care.* CRC, London.
2   Woodman CBJ, Richardson J, and Spence M (1997) Why do we continue to take unnecessary smears? *Br. J. Gen. Pract.* **47**: 645–6.
3   Lo L and Jordan J (1995) Comparative yield of endocervical and metaplastic cells. *Can. Fam. Phys.* **41**: 1497–502.

13

Cancer of the upper gastrointestinal tract

Background

Epidemiology

- In 1995 there were 17 000 new cases of oesophagogastric cancer, nearly 7000 of these affecting the oesophagus.
- In 1995 there were 6830 new cases of pancreatic carcinoma.
- The highest incidence of all upper gastrointestinal cancers is in the sixth decade, and these cancers are more common in men.
- There is geographical variation – carcinoma of the oesophagus is most common in China, Iran, and the Transkei. The incidence of stomach cancer is high in Japan and Chile.

Identifiable risk factors

- Stomach:
  - pernicious anaemia (atrophic gastritis/achlorhydria) increases the risk fivefold
  - history of partial gastrectomy or gastroenterostomy
  - genetic factors: blood group A, HNPCC (*see* Chapter 4)
  - *Helicobacter pylori* (for gastric lymphoma).
- Oesophagus:

- chronic heartburn; 8-fold increase in risk
- Barrett's oesophagus (metaplastic condition); 30-fold increase in risk of cancer
- tobacco smoking and high alcohol intake
- achalasia
- Patterson–Brown–Kelly syndrome (koilonychia, iron-deficiency anaemia, and oesophageal web).
- Pancreas:
  - cigarette smoking (30% of cancers)
  - hereditary factors (3% of cancers).

Pathology and prognosis

- Cancers of the upper two-thirds of the oesophagus are usually squamous-cell carcinomas; one-third of the cancers in the lower oesophagus are adenocarcinomas, possibly arising from areas of squamous metaplasia (Barrett's oesophagus).
- Ninety-five per cent of stomach cancers are adenocarcinomas.
- Pancreatic tumours are most commonly mucin-producing adenocarcinomas.
- According to a recent series from Leeds, survival of oesophogastric cancer is most likely if the tumour is caught early.[1] Unfortunately, long delays still occur in the diagnosis of patients with such cancers.[2]
- Five-year survival in oesophageal cancers is 5–10%.
- The overall 5-year survival for gastric cancer is 10%. However, early gastric cancer has a good 5-year survival of greater than 70%.
- The outlook for pancreatic cancer is poor, with a five-year survival of less than 5%.

Anatomical distribution

- Just under half of oesophageal cancers arise in the middle third of the oesophagus and a similar number in the lower third. Less than 10% arise in the upper third of the oesophagus.
- For stomach cancer, 60% of tumours occur in the pyloris or antrum, 20–30% in the body of the stomach, and 5–20% at the cardia.
- Thirty per cent of pancreatic tumours arise in the head of the pancreas and are often associated with a dilated common bile duct, 20% arise in the body or the tail of the pancreas, and the remainder are more diffuse in origin.

Treatment overview

- Treatment is dictated by the tumour stage, relying mainly on combinations of surgery and radiotherapy.
- For gastric cancer, radical surgery is the only potentially curative treatment, but, unfortunately, one-third of patients are deemed inoperable after full staging investigations.
- Trials of chemotherapy for gastric cancer are currently under way.
- Pancreaticoduodenectomy (Whipple's procedure) is performed for patients with localised non-metastatic pancreatic cancer. Unfortunately, the long-term survival after such a procedure is under 20%.

Screening for gastric cancer

- Mass population screening for early gastric cancer is common practice in China and Japan. In Japan, with screening and aggressive treatment, the proportion of patients with very 'early' disease has increased to 30–40%, with much better survival rates.
- Although there are no RCTs of gastric cancer screening, an increase in the incidence of early gastric cancer has been reported and partly attributed to the availability of open-access gastroscopy. In one study it was demonstrated that the referral for endoscopy of all patients presenting over the age of 40 with new-onset dyspepsia increased the proportion of potentially curative resections from 20% to 63%.

Symptoms in primary care

- In a series of oesophagogastric cancers, the first symptoms were:[1]

Abdominal or chest pain	28%
Dysphagia	24%
Dyspepsia/indigestion	17%
Symptoms from anaemia	17%
Persistent nausea/vomiting	16%
Anorexia (i.e. rapid satiety and fullness)	16%
Weight loss	12%
Heartburn	4%

Dysphagia

Dysphagia is the most common presenting symptom in oesophageal carcinoma. The onset is often insidious with an initial sensation of solid food sticking. This may be in association with regurgitation, aspiration, and weight loss.

Dyspepsia

- The early symptoms of stomach cancer are often vague ('vague dyspepsia'), i.e. loss of appetite or slight nausea and discomfort after meals in a middle-aged patient. Most significant is dyspepsia that is of new onset, that has changed in character, or that is persistent.
- The prevalence of dyspepsia ranges between 20% and 40% in industrialised countries, and roughly 25% of patients seek medical help.[3]
- Within 1 year 34 patients out of 1000 will seek medical advice with a new onset of dyspepsia.[4] It has been estimated that 1 in 53 patients presenting to their GP with dyspepsia for the first time will have gastric cancer.
- In a systematic review examining the discriminant value of symptoms in patients with dyspepsia, it was found that the following were identified as predictors of organic causes in a primary-care setting:[5]
  - higher age
  - male sex
  - pain at night
  - relief by antacids or food
  - previous history of peptic ulcer disease.

Jaundice

- This is the most common presentation of pancreatic cancer due to extra-hepatic biliary obstruction (with pale stools and dark urine).
- It occurs in half of patients at diagnosis, but less than 25% as an initial manifestation (i.e. most patients with pancreatic cancer give a non-specific history of fatigue, anorexia, and weight loss, *see* Chapter 18).
- Such a presentation is usually associated with small tumours of the pancreatic head and a less-advanced stage of the disease, with greater potential for resection.

Non-acute abdominal complaints

In a cohort study examining non-acute abdominal complaints in general practice, the following conclusions were reached:[6]
- eight clinical items were significantly and independently associated

with the presence of organic disease: male sex, greater age, no specific character to pain, epigastric pain, pain affecting sleep, history of blood in stool, no pain relief after defaecation, and abnormal white cell count.

- five clinical items were significantly and independently associated with the presence of neoplasms: male sex, greater age, no specific character to pain, weight loss, and ESR > 20 mm/h.

Signs: the examination

- Often no signs are manifest in upper gastrointestinal malignancy.
- Pallor due to anaemia.
- Jaundice due to extrahepatic biliary obstruction.
- Abdominal epigastric mass.
- A palpable gallbladder in cancer of the pancreas (Courvoisier's sign) has a sensitivity of 30% and a specificity of 100% for extrahepatic biliary obstruction. Thus, in accord with the rule of SpPin (*see* Appendix 1: 'if a test has sufficiently high specificity, a positive result rules in the disorder'), detecting a gallbladder by palpation may be useful in adding further evidence to a diagnostic problem. However, in view of the lower sensitivity, a negative result cannot be used in symptomatic patients to rule out pancreatic cancer as a cause for the jaundice.
- The majority of other signs elicited will be late manifestations of disease (e.g. ascites, hepatomegaly, and supraclavicular lymphadenopathy). Pancreatic cancer is commonly associated with hepatic metastases at diagnosis.

Investigations

- A full blood count and faecal occult blood (FOB) testing may suggest upper gastrointestinal bleeding. It is important to appreciate that examination of the upper gastrointestinal tract can reveal significant abnormalities in 27–43% of patients with positive FOB and negative colonoscopy[7] (*see also* Chapter 4).
- Abnormal liver function tests may suggest metastatic disease but lack adequate sensitivity and specificity to act as screening tests for hepatic metastases in patients with any cancer. A raised serum alkaline phosphatase has a sensitivity and specificity of about 65% for hepatic metastases.
- Ultrasonography has a sensitivity of about 70% and a specificity of about 85% for the detection of pancreatic masses.
- Open-access endoscopy reduces delays in diagnosis if is used appropriately.

- In general, any patient over the age of 45 with recent onset of dyspeptic symptoms or change in dyspeptic symptoms warrants an urgent endoscopy. Patients under the age of 45 with significant symptoms or signs (e.g. vomiting, weight loss, anaemia, or previous gastric surgery; *see* pp. 103–105) may also warrant an urgent endoscopy.

Local referral patterns

- It is very important to check on local arrangements and guidelines for open-access endoscopy and upper abdominal ultrasound investigations.
- If in doubt about the preferred local approach (e.g. for dysphagia), direct contact should be made with the appropriate upper gastrointestinal surgeon.

General sources of information

Cancer Research Campaign (1995) *Stomach Cancer – UK.* Cancer Research Campaign, London.

O'Byrne K and Steward WP (1998) The current status and treatment of pancreatic cancer. *Cancer Top.* **10**: 14–16.

Panzer RJ, Black ER, and Griner PF (1991) *Diagnostic Strategies for Common Medical Problems.* ACP, Philadelphia.

References

1 Martin IG, Young S, Sue-Ling H, and Johnston D (1997) Delays in the diagnosis of oesophagogastric cancer: a consecutive case series. *BMJ* **314**: 467–71.

2 Mikulin T and Hardcastle JD (1987) Gastric cancer – delay in diagnosis and its causes. *Eur. J. Cancer Clin. Oncol.* **23**: 1683–90.

3 Stanghellini V, Tosetti C, Barbara G *et al.* (1998) Management of dyspeptic patients by general practitioners and specialists. *Gut* **43** (Suppl. 1): S21–S23.

4 Meineche-Schmidt V and Krag E (1998) Dyspepsia in general practice in Denmark. A one-year analysis of consulters in general practice. *Scand. J. Prim. Hlth Care* **16**: 216–21.

5 Muris JWM, Starmans R, Pop P *et al.* (1994) Discriminant value of symptoms in patients with dyspepsia. *J. Fam. Pract.* **38**: 139–43.

6 Muris JWM, Starmans R, Fijten GH *et al.* (1995) Non-acute abdominal complaints in general practice: diagnostic value of signs and symptoms. *Br. J. Gen. Pract.* **45**: 313–16.

7 Itzkowitz SH (1998) Heads or tails in a positive faecal occult blood test. *Lancet* **352**: 1490.

14

Haematological malignancies

Section 1: Leukaemia

Background

Epidemiology

- In 1995, there were 5900 new cases of leukaemia in the UK. There are four main types: acute lymphoblastic leukaemia (ALL), acute myeloid leukaemia (AML), chronic lymphocytic leukaemia (CLL), and chronic myeloid leukaemia (CML).

	ALL	AML	CML	CLL
Proportions of leukaemias registered in the UK in 1989	12%	30%	14%	30%
Age distribution	40% occur in 3–5 age group, 85% in individuals under age 15	Most common in children under 4 or adults over 40, 80% in adults over 15	Adults between ages 30 and 60	Mainly adults over age 60

- The overall incidence of all types is 10 per 100 000 per annum.
- Males are more commonly affected than females.
- ALL is the most common leukaemia in childhood.
- AML is the most common leukaemia in adults.

Identifiable risk factors

- Genetic: Down's syndrome, increased incidence in twins.
- Radiation exposure (AML), e.g. radiography in pregnancy, ankylosing spondylitis.
- Chromosomal translocations (Philadelphia chromosome in CML).
- Viral infection, e.g. human T-cell lymphotrophic virus infection in rare T-cell variant CLL.
- Chemicals, e.g. cytotoxic drugs (AML), benzene.
- Smoking (doubles the risk for myeloid leukaemias).
- The vast majority of leukaemias have **no** clear association with any risk factor.

Pathology and prognosis

Acute leukaemias

- ALL:
  - large immature lymphoblasts infiltrate the bone marrow and, occasionally, other sites such as the CNS (causing meningeal irritation) and the testes
  - childhood ALL has a good prognosis, with a 70% 5-year survival rate.
- AML:
  - as in ALL, bone marrow infiltration occurs; other sites of infiltration include liver or spleen, skin and gums
  - overall about 40% of patients are cured of AML.
- Poor prognostic features in acute leukaemias:
  - increasing age (over 40)
  - male sex
  - high leucocyte levels at diagnosis
  - cytogenic abnormalities
  - CNS involvement at diagnosis.

Chronic leukaemias

- CML:
  - the disease is characterised by a chronic phase and randomly occurring blast crises in which the disease transforms into an acute leukaemia (poorly responsive to treatment)
  - blast crises are the major cause of death
  - CML has a median survival of 3–4 years.
- CLL:
  - the disease is insidious with a long natural history
  - 25% of patients may be asymptomatic, with the diagnosis being made incidentally
  - the median survival is 8–10 years, with many patients dying from other causes.

Treatment overview

The management of leukaemia is complex and under constant review. However, some general comments can be made.

Acute leukaemias

- Specific chemotherapy and radiotherapy are given to induce remission, consolidate remission and maintain remission. In addition, supportive treatment may be required to address problems related to bone marrow failure, e.g. anaemia, bleeding, and infection.
- Bone marrow transplantation has a role in the management of both AML and ALL.

Chronic leukaemias

- CML is usually treated with single-dose chemotherapy, such as busulphan.
- In CLL treatment is mainly considered for symptoms, e.g. bone marrow failure. The common choice is oral therapy using chlorambucil or cyclophosphamide.

Prevention

There is no evidence in favour of screening for leukaemia; however, primary prevention for acute leukaemias can be practised by avoiding the use of radiation during pregnancy.

Symptoms and signs in primary care

Symptoms and signs	ALL	AML	CML	CLL
Due to bone marrow failure				
Anaemia (e.g. resulting in malaise, lethargy, dyspnoea, or angina)	+	+	+	+
Thrombocytopenia with bruises or bleeding (e.g. epistaxis, haematuria, or haemoptysis)	+	+	+	+
Leucopenia with signs of infection (e.g. oropharyngeal or chest signs)	+	+	+	+
Generalised symptoms				
Weight loss	+	+	+	+
Fever	+	+	+	+
Sweats	+	+	+	+
Bone pain	+	+	+	+
Splenomegaly	+	+	+++	+
Hepatomegaly	+	+	+	+
Lymphadenopathy	++	+	+	+
Other features of note		Gum hypertrophy	Headaches or confusion due to hyperviscosity; itching	25% asymptomatic

+, May be present; ++, common; +++, very significant.

In children acute leukaemia is usually associated with symptoms of fever, malaise, anorexia, weakness, bleeding, and intractable infection. However, the onset can mimic many other conditions and may be very insidious with irritability and vague aches and pains.

The clinical assessment of lymphadenopathy

See section 2, 'Lymphoma'.

The clinical assessment of splenomegaly

- The size of the spleen can be assessed by inspection, percussion, or palpation.
- The routine examination for splenomegaly by palpation has a sensitivity of 27%, i.e. in accordance with the rule of SnNout (*see* Appendix 1). Failure to detect splenic enlargement cannot definitely rule out splenomegaly.
- Spleen palpation has a higher discriminating ability (87% compared to 55%) in patients already selected as a result of dullness on percussion.
- In primary-care settings, if the possibility of missing splenic enlargement remains an important clinical concern, ultrasonography is indicated.

Investigations in primary care

- Full blood count results: the following findings **may** be present:

	Acute leukaemias	*CML*	*CLL*
RBC	Normochromic, normocytic anaemia	Normochromic, normocytic anaemia	Normochromic, normocytic anaemia
WBC	$1 \times 10^9/l$–$500 \times 10^9/l$ (typically $< 100 \times 10^9/l$)	$100 \times 10^9/l$ $1000 \times 10^9/l$	$50 \times 10^9/l$ $200 \times 10^9/l$
Platelets	Decreased	Decreased (may sometimes be normal or increased)	Decreased
Film	Blast cells and primitive cells	Metamyelocytes and other granulocyte precursors	Small, round lymphocytes

- Following referral, a large number of other investigations may be undertaken, e.g. biochemistry, bone marrow examination, chest radiography, abdominal ultrasound, and coagulation studies.

Follow-up and detection of recurrence

- Once the diagnosis of leukaemia has been made, the further management and follow-up takes place under the care of an appropriate haematologist.
- It is important to check on local arrangements and possibilities for shared care for CLL.
- Local referral patterns and sources of advice should be known in order to deal effectively with any side-effects of treatment or signs of recurrence which may present initially to the general practitioner.

General sources of information

Cancer Research Campaign (1995) *Leukaemia – UK*. Cancer Research Campaign, London.

Grover SA, Barkun AN, and Sackett DL (1993) Does this patient have splenomegaly? *JAMA* **270**: 2218–21.

Section 2: Lymphoma

Background

Epidemiology

- The lymphomas are a diverse group of malignancies, with non-Hodgkin's lymphoma being more common than Hodgkin's disease (7000 compared to 1400 cases per annum in the UK).
- In Hodgkin's disease there is a bimodal age distribution, with peak incidences at 20–24 years and 80–84 years.

Identifiable risk factors

- No clear risk factor for Hodgkin's disease has yet been identified.
- Non-Hodgkin's lymphoma has a number of identifiable risk factors:
  - infectious agents, e.g. *Helicobacter pylori* and gastric lymphoma, Epstein–Barr virus and Burkitt's lymphoma.
  - immunosuppression, e.g. a history of organ transplantation
  - genetic factors, i.e. occasional family clustering, coeliac disease and intestinal lymphoma
  - agrochemicals and petrochemicals.

Pathology and prognosis

The pathological classification is complex and confusing. A simplified approach is shown in Figure 14.1.

Figure 14.1 A simplified approach to the pathological classification of lymphoma.

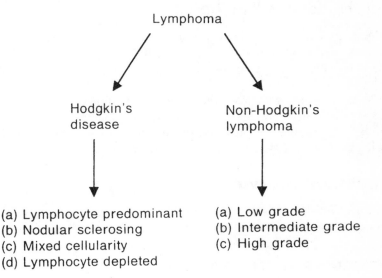

Lymphoma

Hodgkin's disease

Non-Hodgkin's lymphoma

(a) Lymphocyte predominant
(b) Nodular sclerosing
(c) Mixed cellularity
(d) Lymphocyte depleted

(a) Low grade
(b) Intermediate grade
(c) High grade

Hodgkin's disease

- Usually found in lymph nodes, spleen, and liver.
- Commonly, initial involvement is in cervical lymph nodes with incremented involvement of adjacent nodes.
- The staging of Hodgkin's disease follows the Ann Arbor staging system:

Stage I	Disease in a single lymph-node region
Stage II	Disease in two or more regions on the same side of the diaphragm
Stage III	Disease in lymph-node regions on both sides of the diaphragm
Stage IV	Diffuse or disseminated disease in one or more extralymphatic sites (e.g. liver, spleen, skin, bone marrow)

- Each stage is further classified 'A' or 'B' according to the presence of 'B' symptoms, *see* p. 114.

- The 5-year survival rates are reasonably good, for example:

Stage	Five-year survival (%)
IA	90%
IIA	70%

Non-Hodgkin's lymphoma

- Represents a heterogeneous group of disorders in which there is monoclonal proliferation of lymphoid cells.
- Dissemination is widespread and there is no pattern of incremental spread.
- As for Hodgkin's disease, the prognosis and treatment is, to some extent, dictated by the Ann Arbor staging system. Additional prognostic factors are provided by the International Prognostic Index, e.g. age and level of serum lactate dehydrogenase.

Treatment overview

Treatment by chemotherapy and radiotherapy continues to evolve and, in view of its complexity, is primarily the province of oncologists.

Symptoms in primary care

- Painless enlarged lymph nodes (typically in neck in Hodgkin's disease but may be in axilla or groin in non-Hodgkin's). This is the most frequent presenting symptom, occurring in 78% of patients.
- The classical 'B' symptoms characteristic of lymphomas are fever, weight loss (> 10% of body weight over 6 months), and night sweats.
- A recent survey amongst 1034 members of the 'Hodgkin's disease and lymphoma association' revealed that, aside from lymphadenopathy, the most frequent presenting symptoms were:[1]

Symptom	Percentage of patients
Fatigue	24
Drenching night sweats	12
Weight loss	11
Pruritis	11
Breathlessness	11
Pain on drinking alcohol	11

- While moderate nocturnal sweating is common in anxiety states, drenching sweats often require several changes of nightclothes and sheets.
- In some 15–20% of patients with non-Hodgkin's lymphoma, the presentation is in internal groups of lymph nodes (e.g. para-aortic, with back pain) or extralymphatic. Extralymphatic presentation will reflect the tissues involved, with the gastrointestinal system being the most common primary extranodal site. CNS involvement may present with focal neurological signs or features of raised intracranial pressure (*see* Chapter 16).

Signs: the examination

- Lymphadenopathy is common in family practice and has an extensive differential diagnosis, e.g. infectious, autoimmune, iatrogenic hypersensitivity, neoplastic, and a variety of other diseases such as sarcoidosis.[2]
- The incidence of malignancy in patients presenting with unexplained lymphadenopathy to family physicians is very low (1–2%).[3]
- In lymphoma, enlarged lymph nodes are firm, 'rubbery' and usually painless (different from 'craggy' nodes of carcinoma).
- In Hodgkin's disease, there is localised or limited lymphadenopathy.
- In non-Hodgkin's lymphoma, there is limited or generalised lymphadenopathy.
- The presence of lymphadenopathy with splenomegaly (*see* section 1, 'Leukaemia') is compatible with:
  - infectious mononucleosis
  - Hodgkin's disease
  - non-Hodgkin's lymphoma
  - chronic lymphocytic leukaemia.
- The following approach has been suggested when confronted by a patient with lymph node enlargement in primary care, as lymphadenopathy in a primary-care setting is only rarely due to serious disease:[4,5]
  - signs and symptoms rather than lists of 'possible' diagnosis should direct laboratory evaluation
  - if the cause of lymphadenopathy is not evident on initial evaluation, a waiting period of 2–4 weeks is likely to be safe and cost-effective.

Investigations in primary care

- Full blood count: the full blood count may be normal. Occasionally there will be a mild anaemia and a leucocytosis.
- Plain chest radiograph: this can yield valuable information on mediastinal and hilar nodes and the lung fields.

- The diagnosis of lymphoma ultimately rests entirely on biopsy of a lymph node or an affected extranodal site by an appropriately trained surgeon.

Follow-up and detection of recurrence

- Once the diagnosis of lymphoma has been made, the further investigation, management, and follow-up takes place under the care of an appropriate oncologist.
- It is important to check on local arrangements and possibilities for shared care.
- Local referral patterns and sources of advice should be known in order to deal effectively with any side-effects of treatment or signs of recurrence which may present initially to the general practitioner.

General sources of information

Cancer Research Campaign (1997) *Non-Hodgkin's Lymphoma in Adults – UK*. Cancer Research Campaign, London.

References

1 RCGP Connection (1996) GP fact file lymphomas. *RCGP Connection* **83**: 6.
2 Pangalis GA, Vassilakopoulos TP, Boussiotis VA, and Fessas P (1993) Clinical approach to lymphadenopathy. *Semin. Oncol.* **20**: 570–82.
3 Fijten GH and Blijham GH (1988) Unexplained lymphadenopathy in family practice. An evaluation of the probability of malignant causes and the effectiveness of physicians' workup. *J. Fam. Pract.* **27**: 373–6.
4 Allhiser JN, McKnight TA, and Shank JC (1981) Lymphadenopathy in a family practice. *J. Fam. Pract.* **12**: 27–32.
5 Williamson HA (1985) Lymphadenopathy in a family practice: a descriptive study of 249 cases. *J. Fam. Pract.* **20**: 449–52.

Section 3: Multiple myeloma

Background

Epidemiology

- In 1995, 3450 new cases of myeloma were registered in the UK.
- The peak incidence is between the ages of 60 and 70.
- It is more common in Africans than Caucasians.

Identifiable risk factors

None evident.

Pathology and prognosis

- Multiple myeloma is a malignant disorder of the plasma cells, producing monoclonal paraproteins.
- Myeloma is classified according to the type of paraprotein produced – most are IgG (55%), other main types are IgA (21%) and light chains only (22%).
- The atypical plasma cells infiltrate the bone marrow, resulting in bone marrow failure and local bone destruction.
- There is a long preclinical phase (often up to 20–25 years) and the disorder may be discovered incidentally.
- Poor prognostic features at diagnosis are significant anaemia and thrombocytopenia, plasma-cell leukaemia, renal failure, and hypoalbuminaemia.

Treatment overview

Some asymptomatic patients may simply be monitored. Others may require supportive treatment to preserve renal function (e.g. fluids, management of hypercalcaemia and hyperuricaemia) and specific chemotherapy or radiotherapy.

Symptoms and signs in primary care

- Clinical features may be few or non-specific, e.g. pallor and tiredness due to anaemia.
- Bone pain (especially in the back and chest) is present in two-thirds of new patients with myeloma.
- Bone destruction may result in pathological fractures or neurological complications (e.g. nerve root or spinal cord compression in 5–10% of patients).
- Fifteen per cent of patients may exhibit hepatomegaly.
- Hyperviscosity and hypercalcaemia can cause confusion.
- Impaired immune function may increase susceptibility to infection.

Investigations

- FBC: in 60% of patients there may be normochromic, normocytic anaemia.
- Biochemistry: in up to half the patients there may be evidence of renal dysfunction; in one-third, hypercalcaemia.
- ESR and plasma viscosity: these will be abnormal in 90% of patients.
- Protein electrophoresis: paraprotein band.
- Urinalysis: Bence Jones protein.
- Plain radiographs may reveal lytic lesions, osteoporosis, or fractures.

Diagnosis, follow-up, and detection of recurrence

- The key diagnostic triad for myeloma consists of serum or urinary M protein, increased number of bone marrow plasma cells, and osteolytic lesions.
- The main conditions to consider in the differential diagnosis are monoclonal gammopathy of undetermined significance (MGUS), primary amyloidosis, and metastatic carcinoma.
- Once the diagnosis of multiple myeloma has been made, the further management and follow-up takes place under the care of an appropriate haematologist.
- It is important to check on local arrangements and possibilities for shared care.
- Local referral patterns and sources of advice should be known in order to deal effectively with any side-effects of treatment or signs of deterioration which may present initially to the general practitioner.

General sources of information

Weatherall DJ, Ledingham JGG, and Warrell DA (eds) (1996) *Oxford Textbook of Medicine*, Vol. 3. Oxford University Press, Oxford.

15

Head and neck cancer

There are a number of head and neck cancers (many of which are very rare). This chapter restricts itself primarily to the oral cancers (lip, tongue, and mouth) and laryngeal cancer.

Background

Epidemiology

- Each year in the UK there are over 2500 cases of oral cancer and about 1400 people die of the disease.
- More than 90% of oral cancers occur in patients over the age of 45, with the incidence increasing steadily until the age of 65. They are twice as common amongst men than women.
- Cancers of the larynx are most common between the ages of 50 and 70.

Identifiable risks factors

- Smoking tobacco.
- Heavy alcohol consumption.
- Chewing tobacco, oral snuff or betel quid (Asians) (oral cancers).
- Sun exposure (lip cancer).

Other suggested risk factors

- Poor oral hygiene.
- Long-standing dental trauma or infection.
- Dietary deficiencies of vitamins A and C and iron.

Anatomical distribution of oral cancers

- Ninety per cent arise in the floor of the mouth, the side of the tongue, the lingual sulcus (grooves at the sides of the tongue), or behind the teeth.
- Cancers related to chewing tobacco or betel quid may arise in the cheek and at the junction of the lower and upper lips.

Pathology and prognosis

- Ninety per cent of oral and laryngeal cancers are squamous-cell carcinomas.

Oral cancers

- Although easily detected and often cured in their early stages, most oral cancers are moderately advanced at the time of diagnosis, i.e. oral cancers have a low 5-year survival rate (52%). Early cancers of the lip and oral cavity are highly curable.
- People at risk from oral cancer are more likely to visit their GP than their dentist and yet most physicians believe dentists are primarily responsible for detecting oral cancer.[1]
- Most patients with oral cancer have been found to delay seeking professional advice for more than 3 months after becoming aware of an oral sign or symptom.

Laryngeal cancers

- Survival in patients with laryngeal cancer is dependent on the stage and site of the tumour.
- Cancer of the larynx does not readily metastasise to distant parts of the body and if local eradication of the disease is achieved, then a permanent cure is very likely.

- The majority of early tumours can be treated successfully with 5-year survival rates in excess of 75%.
- Advanced tumours have a much poorer prognosis (less than 30% at 5 years following radical and mutilating surgery).
- According to Hoare *et al.*, early diagnosis based on symptoms is feasible in the majority of cases.[2]

Treatment overview

Radiotherapy and surgery are the main treatment methods for all head and neck cancers.

Screening for oral cancer

There is insufficient evidence to establish that population screening would result in a decrease in mortality from oral cancer.[3,4]

Symptoms in primary care

Oral cancers

- Most patients are asymptomatic.
- Ulceration of oral tumours may result in soreness.
- Occasional cervical lymphadenopathy may be noticed as a lump in the head or neck.

Laryngeal cancers[5]

- Hoarseness (lasting for more than 4 weeks) is the most common symptom as most laryngeal cancers involve the vocal chords. This is particularly significant in patients over the age of 50 who smoke and drink heavily.
- Other common symptoms are muffled voice, dysphagia, and pain in the throat, neck, or ear.
- Occasional cervical lymphadenopathy may be noticed as a lump in the head or neck.

Signs: the examination

- Leukoplakia (whitish) and erythroplastic (reddish) lesions are the earliest signs of squamous-cell carcinoma of the mouth. Often an oral cancer is preceded by several months of these visible precancerous lesions.
- Any oral ulcer or lesion that persists for more than 4 weeks should be taken seriously.
- Cervical lymphadenopathy may be identified.

Local referral patterns

- Obvious oral cancers or patients with persistent oral lesions need to be referred to an appropriate oral or maxillofacial surgeon.
- Patients with persistent hoarseness or other suspicious symptoms need to be referred to an appropriate ear, nose, and throat surgeon.
- It is essential to be clear about local referral arrangements operating in your area.

General sources of information

Cancer Registry Special Report Series (1994) *Head and Neck Cancers*. Yorkshire Cancer Organisation, Leeds.
Cancer Research Campaign (1993) *Oral Cancer*. Cancer Research Campaign, London.

References

1 Goodman HS, Yellowitz JA, and Horowitz AM (1995) Oral cancer prevention. The role of family practitioners. *Arch. Fam. Med.* **4**: 628–36.
2 Hoare TJ, Thomson HG, and Proops DW (1993) Detection of laryngeal cancer – the case for early specialist assessment. *J. R. Soc. Med.* **86**: 390–2.
3 Sprangler JG (1995) Open your mouth and say, 'ahhh...'. Oral cancer screening and family physicians. *Arch. Fam. Med.* **4**: 585–6.
4 Jullien JA, Zakrzewska JM, Downer MC, and Speight PM (1995) Attendance and compliance at an oral cancer screening programme in general medical practice. *Oral. Oncol., Eur. J. Cancer* **31B**: 202–6.
5 McKenna JP, Leonard RJ, Fornatara-Clerici LM, and McMenamin PG (1991) Laryngeal cancer: diagnosis, treatment and speech rehabilitation. *Arch. Fam. Pract.* **44**: 123–9.

16

Central nervous system tumours

Background

Epidemiology

- In 1995, 3910 new central nervous system tumours were diagnosed in the UK.
- Brain tumours are the most common solid neoplasms in children.
- With the exception of meningiomas, brain tumours are more common in men than in women.

Identifiable risk factors

- Genetic predisposition, e.g. associations with neurofibromatosis and tuberous sclerosis.
- Immunosuppression (lymphomas, *see* Chapter 14).

Pathology and prognosis

- Gliomas account for half of the primary CNS tumours; meningiomas, one-quarter. Pituitary craniopharyngiomas and adenomas account for one-fifth.

- Twenty per cent of all cerebral tumours are metastatic, with nearly half of these originating from pulmonary primaries.
- Direct infiltration is the main mode of spread for all primary cerebral tumours.
- The 5-year survival of low-grade glioma is 50% following surgical treatment.

Treatment overview

- Management generally consists of some form of surgical intervention, often combined with radiotherapy and, occasionally, chemotherapy. There are five potential goals of surgery: to establish a diagnosis, to remove the tumour, to improve symptoms, to prolong life, to increase the sensitivity of the tumour to other forms of treatment.
- It is important to appreciate that this therapeutic area is changing rapidly, with the addition of newer techniques such as computer-directed surgery, radiosurgery, brachytherapy, and hyperthermia.

Symptoms and signs in primary care

A characteristic clinical feature of all intracranial neoplasms is that they produce **progressive symptoms**. The rate of progression varies from an acute apoplectic onset to gradual mental deterioration.

Raised intracranial pressure

This produces generalised symptoms which may lead to the following:
- Non-specific symptoms (i.e. irritability, lethargy or withdrawn behaviour, decreased appetite and vomiting) are, more than half of the time, the only findings present at diagnosis of a brain tumour in an infant or child. Mental changes constitute a frequent general clinical manifestation in adults. They are often subtle in presentation and typically the onset may pass unnoticed, even by close relatives or friends, until a particularly unusual behaviour occurs. Psychomotor retardation (i.e. emotional lability, inertia, faulty insight, and forgetfulness) is the most common mental change.
- Headaches: these occur in about 50% of patients at some time during the course of the illness. There are many causes of new-onset, recurrent headaches but, according to Seller,[1] organic brain disease should be suspected if one or more of the following symptoms are noted:
  - intermittent or continuous headache that progressively increases in frequency and severity (i.e. a change in character of the headache)

- headache that is exacerbated by coughing or straining at stool
- headache that is worse in the morning
- vomiting
- headache that disturbs sleep
- onset of severe headaches after age 50.

In young children, transient resolution of headaches may occur due to spreading of the sutures, which temporarily accommodates the increase in pressure for a short period.
- Examination may reveal:
  - papilloedema
  - reduced level of consciousness
  - an enlarging head circumference in a child
  - double vision due to a VI nerve palsy (false localising sign).

Practical considerations (papilloedema)

- The normal optic disc is circular and rosy-pink in colour, although slightly paler than the surrounding retina. In the early stages of papilloedema, the disc is pinker than normal.
- Subsequently, there is blurring of the disc margins (often the nasal edge blurs before the temporal edge).
- Later the disc swelling lifts the surface of the disc above the level of the surrounding retina, i.e. veins appear congested and tortuous, flame-shaped haemorrhages and white exudate may be seen.

According to Shapiro,[2] currently less than 20% of patients with intracranial tumours have papilloedema.

Neurological effects: new-onset epilepsy

- Seizures occurring for the first time in adults are more likely to be due to focal cerebral disease, especially neoplasms.
- Seizures, both generalised and focal, occur in 35% of patients with cerebral tumours.
- Metastatic tumours are less likely to induce seizures than are primary brain tumours.

Specific symptoms

- Focal manifestations of intracranial tumours depend on the effect on specific areas of the brain, for example:

- disturbances of vision may occur in half of pituitary tumours (initially these are often temporary and unilateral); there may also be symptoms and signs of hyperprolactinaemia
- unilateral disturbance of hearing, unilateral tinnitus and vertigo may occur with acoustic neuromas
- cerebellar tumours may produce incoordination.
- False localising signs (i.e. suggesting a location of a specific lesion due to prolonged elevation of intracranial pressure) are more common in slowly growing neoplasms such as meningiomas.

Investigations and local referral patterns

- Specific radiological investigations must be employed to confirm the diagnosis of the brain tumour, its location, and to rule out other diagnoses.
- Routine skull radiographs have limited usefulness in the diagnosis of brain tumours. They may demonstrate evidence of chronically raised intracranial pressure (erosion of the dorsum sellae, split sutures in infants), the presence of abnormal calcifications, or enlargement of the sella turcica. Osteolytic or osteoblastic metastases may be visible in the skull vault.
- Magnetic resonance imaging (MRI) demonstrates the normal anatomy of the brain better than does a CT scan. The addition of gadolinium enhancement has made MRI the procedure of choice in diagnosing brain tumours.
- It is important to be familiar with the local referral patterns used in your area for adults and children with symptoms or signs suggestive of intracranial tumours.

General sources of information

Bannister R (1978) *Brain's Clinical Neurology*. Oxford University Press, Oxford.
Robertson PL (1998) Pediatric brain tumors. *Primary Care* **25**: 323–39.

References

1 Seller RH (1996) *Differential Diagnosis of Common Complaints*. WB Saunders, Toronto.
2 Shapiro WR, Shapiro JR, and Walker RW (1995) Central nervous system. In: MD Abeldoff, JO Armitage, AS Lichter, and JE Niederhuber (eds) *Clinical Oncology*. Churchill Livingstone, New York.

17

Skin cancer

Section 1: Basal- and squamous-cell carcinomas

Background

Epidemiology

- Basal- (BCC) and squamous-cell (SCC) carcinomas of the skin are probably the most common malignancies.
- It is estimated that the incidence rate for basal cell carcinoma is 40 000 new diagnoses per annum in the UK.
- Around 10 000 squamous cell carcinomas are diagnosed annually in the UK.
- There are 400 deaths per year, mainly due to squamous-cell carcinoma.
- Basal-cell carcinoma has a peak incidence at age 60–80 years.

Identifiable risk factors

- Chronic sun exposure and history of sunburn.
- Fair skin, light hair, light eyes.
- Poor ability to tan.
- Exposure to ionising radiation (e.g. previous irradiation).

- Family history: there is a general familial risk as well as associations with specific syndromes, e.g. xeroderma pigmentosum or Gorlin's syndrome (a dominantly inherited form of BCC occurring mainly under the age of 40).
- Personal history of skin cancer.
- Scarred or traumatised skin for squamous-cell carcinoma (e.g. chronic varicose (Marjolin's) ulcers, burn scars, cutaneous tuberculosis, sinuses from chronic oesteomyelitis and epidermolysis bullosa).
- Arsenic treatment.
- The common precursor lesions for invasive non-mucosal squamous-cell carcinoma are actinic keratoses and Bowen's disease (squamous-cell carcinoma *in situ*).

Pathology and prognosis

- Squamous-cell carcinoma is graded 1–4 depending on the proportion of differentiating cells present, the degree of atypia of the tumour cells, and depth of tumour penetration. The lesions can occur in several forms; Bowen's disease is *in situ* squamous-cell carcinoma.
- Basal-cell carcinomas and squamous-cell carcinomas tend to be locally invasive but can become secondarily infected.
- Five per cent of squamous-cell carcinomas spread to regional lymph nodes; 0.1% of basal-cell carcinomas spread to regional lymph nodes.
- The risk of metastasis with squamous-cell carcinoma depends on the degree of differentiation, depth of penetration, and the location of the lesion – squamous-cell carcinomas of the lip or ear have a higher risk for metastasis.
- Squamous cell carcinomas that arise in areas of skin that are not exposed to the sun generally have a poorer prognosis.
- If either cancer is detected and treated early, the prognosis is excellent with cure rates above 95%.

Treatment overview

For both basal-cell carcinoma of the skin and squamous-cell carcinoma the traditional methods of treatment involve the use of cryosurgery, radiation therapy, electrodissection and curettage, and simple excision.

Clinical presentations

Basal-cell carcinoma

- Although there are many different clinical presentations for basal-cell carcinoma, the most characteristic type is the asymptomatic nodular or nodular ulcerative lesion.
- The typical presentation is in the form of a papule that is elevated from the surrounding skin, has a shiny, pearly quality with overlying telangiectasia.
- Other presentations include an enlarged, flat plaque with a pearly edge, a non-healing scabbing erosion or ulcer, or a pigmented papule.
- Classic features may be absent and the diagnosis of any suspicious skin lesion should be confirmed by biopsy.
- Basal-cell carcinomas are very rare in non-hair bearing skin, are often multiple, and are frequently associated with changes of solar damage, e.g. keratoses.

Squamous-cell carcinoma

- The classical appearance is nodular, or nodular with central ulceration or ulcerated with raised everted nodular edge. If the hyperkeratotic scale is removed, the tumour will often bleed.
- It is often more difficult to be certain of the diagnosis of SCC without biopsy than BCC.
- Any sore that does not heal should be treated with suspicion. A sore that does not heal after 2–3 months has a predictive value for skin cancer of 2–4% in primary-care populations.[1]
- As in the case of BCCs, squamous-cell carcinomas tend to occur on exposed portions of the skin; however, squamous-cell carcinomas of areas of skin not exposed to the sun are important to identify since they have a greater tendency to metastasise.
- Actinic keratoses are red, scaly patches that arise on areas of chronically sun-exposed skin. It is thought that as many as 5% of actinic keratoses will evolve into the locally invasive carcinoma.
- Bowen's disease (squamous-cell carcinoma *in situ*) usually presents as a single, red, well-demarcated, thin plaque that ranges in size from a few millimetres to several centimetres. Of these, 3–5% will develop into squamous-cell carcinomas with a high potential for metastasis.

Practical considerations[2]

- Examination of the skin requires good lighting and, if possible, the assistance of a magnifying lens.
- It is often helpful to touch and manipulate the skin as well as looking at it.
- Total-body examination should be considered in all patients with a history of non-melanocytic skin cancer (NMSC), to check for second primaries.

Follow-up

- Fifty per cent of patients treated for basal- and squamous-cell carcinoma will have another skin cancer in 5 years; therefore it is important for regular, life-long surveillance to be instituted.[3]
- Persons with a history of NMSC are at increased risk of cancer mortality, i.e. it is necessary to be alert for certain non-cutaneous cancers as well.[4]
- The melanoma risk is increased 3–17% if there has been a previous squamous-cell carcinoma or basal-cell carcinoma.
- Actinic keratosis is a premalignant condition that should be referred for appropriate treatment
- It is important to check on the follow-up arrangements recommended in your area for NMSCs.

Local referral patterns

- All skin lesions removed by general practitioners should be submitted for pathological examination to establish the precise diagnosis (see p. 137).
- It is important to be familiar with local arrangements for dealing with patients with suspected NMSC quickly and efficiently.

General sources of information

British Association of Dermatologists (1996) *Providing Cutaneous Oncology Services.* British Association of Dermatologists, London.
Callen JP (1978) Squamous cell carcinoma of the skin. *Primary Care* **5**: 299–311.
Marghoob AA (1997) Basal and squamous cell carcinomas. What every primary care physician should know. *Postgrad. Med.* **102**: 139–54.

Stawiski MA (1978) Basal cell carcinoma. A practical approach to diagnosis and therapy. *Primary Care* **5**: 283–98.

References

1   Holtedahl KA (1989) *Diagnosis of cancer in general practice.* MD Thesis, University of Tromso.
2   Brodland DG (1995) Diagnosis of nonmelanoma skin cancer. *Clin. Derm.* **13**: 551–7.
3   Kahn HS, Tatham LM, Patel AV *et al.* (1998) Increased cancer mortality following a history of nonmelanoma skin cancer. *JAMA* **280**: 910–12.
4   Frisch M, Hjalgrim H, Olsen JH, and Melbye M (1996) Risk for subsequent cancer after diagnosis of basal-cell carcinoma. A population-based, epidemiological study. *Ann. Int. Med.* **125**: 815–21.

Section 2: Melanoma

Background

Epidemiology

- In 1995 there were nearly 5000 new cases of melanoma in the UK (3000 of these were in women).
- Eighteen per cent of melanoma cases occur in people aged 15–39 years.
- In women aged 20–35 melanoma is the most common cancer after cervical cancer.
- Melanoma causes 1500 deaths per annum in the UK.
- More common in light-skinned races.

Identifiable risk factors

- Family history of melanoma or dysplastic naevus syndrome.
- Personal history of melanoma.
- History of non-melanocyte skin cancer.
- Tendency to burn or history of prior sunburn.
- Naevi.

Low risk (relative risk <2)

Up to 50 naevi less than 5 mm in diameter.

Moderate risk (relative risk >4)

More than five naevi greater than 5 mm in diameter.

High risk (relative risk >10)

More than 10 dysplastic naevi, i.e. naevi more than 5 mm in diameter with an irregular edge and irregular pigmentation.

Anatomical distribution

- Although most melanomas arise in the skin, they also may arise from mucosal surfaces (e.g. aerodigestive tract, anus, and vagina). Melanoma can also affect the eye – melanoma of choroid.
- Melanoma in women occurs more commonly on the extremities and in men on the trunk or head and neck **but any part** of the skin is a potential site for melanoma development.

Melanoma distribution

Site	Males (%)	Females (%)
Trunk	35	13
Legs	25	56
Arms	17	17
Head and neck	23	14

Pathology and prognosis

Summary of features of the four main types of malignant melanoma

Type of melanoma	Main features	% of cases in United Kingdom
Superficial spreading melanoma	All body areas but most common on the lower legs of younger women and the back and neck in younger men. Potentially of low risk if treated early (radial growth with flat irregular margins)	50–70

Nodular melanoma	All body areas but the trunk is the most common site. A blue/black raised lesion. Grows fairly quickly in a vertical fashion with early metastases and a poor prognosis	15–30
Lentigo maligna melanoma	On light-exposed areas of skin, particularly head and neck in elderly patients. Irregular margins with slow growth.	4–10
Acral or acral–lentiginous melanoma	These are rare, but include melanomas on the palms, soles, and digits, e.g. sub-ungal	2–8

- The prognosis is affected by clinical and histological factors and by the anatomical location of the lesion.
- Melanomas arising on the extremities or in women seem to have a better prognosis.
- Ulcerated melanomas or nodular melanomas are associated with a poorer prognosis.
- The microstage of malignant melanoma is determined by the vertical thickness in millimetres (Breslow's classification) and/or the anatomical level of local invasion (Clark's classification) on histological examination.
- The Breslow stage predicts most accurately the subsequent behaviour of malignant melanoma:

Breslow thickness	Five-year survival (%)
<1.5 mm	93
1.5–3.5 mm	67
>3.5 mm	37

- Because the tumour's thickness at excision is the primary prognostic determinant, early detection through the history and physical examination plays an important role in the patient's course.
- The most common sites for secondary spread are the lungs and the liver.

Treatment overview

- The treatment of localised melanoma is surgical excision with margins proportional to the microstage of the primary lesion.
- Adjuvant chemotherapy has not been shown to increase survival.

- Melanomas are considered to be relatively radioresistant tumours.
- Adjuvant biological therapy, e.g. α-interferon, has been shown to increase disease-free and overall survival for patients with node-positive disease.

Prevention

Overview of melanoma screening by visual inspection of the skin

The disease	Response	Comment
Is it an important problem?	Yes	See p. 131
Is the natural history well understood?	Reasonably	Some evidence of spontaneous regression (up to 1% of cases)
Is there a recognised latent of early stage?	Yes	See p. 133

The test: visual inspection of the skin	Respones	Comment
Is it simple to perform?	Yes	But need to examine the entire skin surface
Is it expensive?	Yes	In New Zealand it is estimated that an annual full-skin examination of adults aged 35–64 by general practitioners would occupy up to 5% of a GPs clinical time
Is it sufficiently accurate?	Unknown	See p. 136. Scoring systems have never been assessed in a primary-care setting
Is it acceptable with adequate compliance?	Unknown	No information available on unnecessary biopsies and anxiety
Are there adequate facilities for the diagnosis and treatment of any abnormalities detected?	No	Relies on existing dermatology and pathology services

The treatment	Response
Is there any effective treatment?	Yes, see p. 133
Does treatment at an earlier stage result in more benefit than treatment started at a later stage?	Results from RCTs are not yet available. There is no unequivocal evidence that earlier detection by screening reduces mortality from melanoma

Selective screening has been suggested for certain groups, e.g. those with dysplastic naevi, a positive family history, fair complexion and light skin, propensity to sunburn, or the presence of a changing mole.

Primary prevention

Individuals are encouraged to reduce excessive sun exposure:

- personal behaviour changes for individuals, e.g. minimizing UV exposure, using sunscreens
- policy and environmental interventions, e.g. provision of shady areas and preservation of ozone layer
- a public education campaign in western Scotland to encourage earlier referral and treatment succeeded in reducing the absolute number of thick tumours and melanoma-related mortality in women.[1]

Clinical features in primary care

- The diagnosis of melanoma, especially early melanoma is difficult.
- A study in Australia revealed that the overall accuracy rate for melanoma was 65.6%; seborrhoeic keratosis, melanocytic naevi, and BCC were the most common clinical misdiagnoses given.[2]
- Early melanomas and thin melanomas are more difficult to diagnose (especially if <6 mm).
- The key decision is whether to biopsy suspicious lesions.
- Two checklists have been developed as diagnostic aids:
  - ABCD (USA)
  (i) if the lesion is bisected, one half is not identical to other half – asymmetry (A)
  (ii) when the border is uneven or ragged as opposed to smooth and straight – border irregularity (B)
  (iii) when more than one shade of pigment is present – colour variegation (C)
  (iv) when the diameter is greater than 6 mm – diameter (D).

A positive result has one or more of these features. Others add in additional historical features, such as a change in pre-existing pigmented naevus or the development of new pigmented lesion. Some scales also add elevation above the skin surface (E).

– UK (revised seven-point checklist)

Major signs
  Change in size
  Change in shape
  Change in colour
Minor signs
  Inflammation
  Crusting or bleeding
  Sensory change
  Diameter >7 mm

One or more major signs – consider rapid referral
Additional presence of one or more minor signs – increased possibility of melanoma
Three or four minor signs without major sign – consider referral

- A scoring system has also been applied to the features on the UK scale, with 2 points for each major criterion and 1 point for each minor. Referral is indicated if there is at least one major sign or a score of 3 points or more.
- The sensitivity and specificity of the two scoring systems have been assessed amongst dermatologists.[3] Unfortunately, the scoring systems have yet to be validated in primary care.

	ABCD (E) (i.e. one out of 5)	ABCD (BCD on checklist)	Seven-point checklist (one major feature)	Seven-point checklist (2 points for major, 1 point for minor, >3)
Sensitivity	92%	100%	100%	79%
Specificity	–	98%	37%	30%

Patients have an important role to play in the early diagnosis of melanoma

- Patients using the seven-point checklist had a specificity of 32% (similar to the 30% for doctors).

- Patients need to be asked about lesions of concern, e.g. new moles or a change in size, shape, colour, or sensation of a pre-existing mole. Over half of all melanomas (especially those that involve a change in size or colour) are discovered by patients.

Investigations

Excision biopsy continues to be undertaken by general practitioners. Recent reviews have emphasised the importance of the following:[4,5]

- because of the uncertainty of clinical diagnosis of pigmented skin lesions all specimens should be submitted for histopathological diagnosis (in the North-East Thames region, GPs underused the pathology service)
- amelanotic tumours are seen in 5% of cases (in a study in the North-East Thames region, tumours excised by GPs were more likely to be amelanotic).
- general practitioners should be confident and appropriately trained in both the diagnostic and technical aspects of excision biopsy (in the North-East Thames study, incomplete excision of melanomas was significantly more likely in the GP group).

Follow-up and detection of recurrence

It is recommended that patients with malignant melanoma are followed up for a minimum of 5 years in order to assess:

- any signs of local or regional recurrence, e.g. regional lymphadeno-pathy and/or lumps under the skin around the scar
- metastatic disease – most common sites are the lungs and liver
- the presence of any other suspicious skin lesions.

Larger lesions (>1.5 cm in diameter at diagnosis) may be followed-up for at least ten years. It is important to check on the local arrangements in your district.

Local referral patterns

- Any patient with a pigmented skin lesion, which could possibly be a malignant melanoma, should be referred urgently to a dermatologist, surgeon, or plastic surgeon with an interest in pigmented lesions and malignant melanoma. Urgent referral for plastic surgery is particularly appropriate for larger lesions (>1 cm in diameter) and cosmetically difficult lesions, i.e. around the eyes or nose.

- All patients who have had lesions removed by general practitioners, which have subsequently been reported as malignant melanomas, should be referred immediately for further assessment to an appropriate specialist (most commonly a plastic surgeon especially if there is evidence of incomplete excision).
- It is important to be familiar with local arrangements for dealing with patients with pigmented lesions quickly and efficiently. Patients with a melanoma or suspected melanoma should ideally be seen by an appropriate specialist within one week. Patients with dysplastic naevi should also be seen rapidly.

General sources of information

Austoker J (1995) *Cancer Prevention in Primary Care*. BMJ Publishing Group, London.

Girgis A, Clarke P, Burton RC, and Sanson-Fisher RW (1996) Screening for melanoma by primary health care physicians: a cost-effectiveness analysis. *J. Med. Screen.* **3**: 47–53.

Johnson N, Mant D, Newton J, and Yudkin PL (1994) Role of primary care in the prevention of malignant melanoma. *Br. J. Gen. Pract.* **44**: 523–6.

Koh HK, Geller AC, Miller DR *et al.* (1996) Prevention and early detection strategies for melanoma and skin cancer. *Arch. Dermatol.* **132**: 436–43.

Roberts D (ed) (1998) *Management of Primary Malignant Melanoma of the Skin. Guidelines for Wales*. Clinical Effectivenes Support Unit, Cardiff.

Whited JD, Hall RP, Simel DL, and Horner RD (1997) Primary care clinicians' performance for detecting actinic keratoses and skin cancer. *Arch. Int. Med.* **157**: 985–90.

References

1 MacKie RM and Hole D (1992) Audit of public education campaign to encourage earlier detection of malignant melanoma. *BMJ* **304**: 1012–15.

2 Mackenzie-Wood AR, Milton GW, and deLauney JW (1998) Melanoma: accuracy of clinical diagnosis. *Aust. J. Derm.* **39**: 31–3.

3 Whited JD and Grichnik JM (1998) Does this patient have a mole or a melanoma? *JAMA* **279**: 696–701.

4 Khorshid SM, Pinney E, and Newton-Bishop JA (1998) Melanoma excision by general practitioners in North-East Thames region, England. *Br. J. Derm.* **138**: 412–17.

5 Bricknell MCM (1993) Skin biopsies of pigmented skin lesions performed by general practitioners and hospital specialists. *Br. J. Gen. Pract.* **43**: 199–201.

Non-specific features of malignant disease

Involuntary weight loss

- The significance of involuntary weight loss should not be underestimated; a number of studies have indicted that underlying pathology can be found in three-quarters of such patients.

Weight loss studies

Study	Thompson and Morris[1]	Rabinovitz et al.[2]	Marton et al.[3]
Number of patients	45 family practice centre patients	154 internal medicine patients	91 male veterans, both inpatient and outpatient
Mean age (year)	72	64	59
Percentage with no cause identified	24%	23%	26%
Percentage diagnosed with cancer	16%	36%	19%

- According to Riefe,[4] malignancy is the most common cause of weight loss, especially when major symptoms and signs are absent.
- Although any cancer may present with weight loss, the gastrointestinal tract (especially the pancreas, *see* Chapter 13) is the most frequent site for occult tumours to be found.

- A weight loss of greater than 5% in 6 months or greater than 10% over 1 year should trigger concern.
- In the study by Marton *et al.*, half of the patients with weight loss had key signs or symptoms pointing to disease at a specific site, e.g. weight loss and cough.[3] Consequently, diagnostic testing should be directed towards areas of concern elicited from the history and examination.
- Weight loss is a predictor of prognosis and response to therapy for a number of cancers. Median survival has been shown to be shorter in cancer patients with weight loss.

Back pain

- Back pain is a common complaint in general practice.
- Although serious underlying disease is rare in patients with back problems, back pain can be the first manifestation of cancer (most commonly from metastatic disease).
- According to Deyo and Diehl,[5] a few key items from the medical history can be used to rule in or rule out cancer:

Features in medical history	Likelihood ratio
Age $\geqslant 50$	2.7
Previous cancer history	14.7
Unexplained weight loss	2.7
Failure to improve with 1 month of therapy	2.6
Bed rest no relief	1.8
Duration of pain >1 month	3.0

- Thus 'high-risk' patients are those with a prior history of cancer. 'Low-risk' patients are those under age 50 with no history of cancer, no weight loss or other sign of systemic illness, and no history of failure to improve with conservative therapy.
- An 'intermediate-risk' group includes patients over age 50, those with failure of conservative therapy, and those with unexplained weight losses or other signs of systemic illness (e.g. lymphadenopathy, haematuria). For this group the ESR (significant level taken to be $\geqslant 20$ mm/h) may be particularly useful in raising or lowering the suspicion of cancer (*see* p. 141).
- The further assessment of patients with 'red flags' involves the use of spinal radiographs to rule out malignancy. However, it is important to appreciate that the sensitivity of plain films is approximately 65–70% (and may be even less sensitive early in the course of the disease).[6] It has therefore been suggested that patients with red flags (especially a

previous cancer history) and negative radiography findings require further work-up. The use of other imaging studies, such as a bone scan, CT, or MRI, may be indicated in such circumstances.

Venous thromboembolism

- Over the past century it has been suggested repeatedly that deep-vein thrombosis may be a predictor of the subsequent diagnosis of cancer. Recently Sorensen *et al.* noted that the standardised incidence ratio for cancer was highest during the first 6 months after hospital admission for either deep-vein thrombosis or pulmonary embolism.[7]
- According to Baron *et al.*, the risk of cancers in the lung and brain, and of certain abdominal and haematological malignant diseases, was especially increased soon after a hospital admission with a thrombotic event. They also noted that younger patients with thromboembolic diagnoses had a higher relative risk of cancer in the year after admission. Furthermore, their data indicated that the association could persist for 10 years after the thrombotic event.[8]
- Although the studies by Baron and Sorensen are subject to bias and confounding, it is important to appreciate that 40–60% of the cancers that appear after venous thromboembolism are not metastatic at the time of detection. Furthermore, decision analysis of screening for occult cancer in patients with idiopathic deep-vein thrombosis has revealed potential gains in life expectancy. Thus, in any patient with primary venous thromboembolism, Buller and Cate[9] suggest the following measured approach:
  - routine clinical history and examination
  - chest radiograph and routine blood tests
  - consideration of mammography and pelvic ultrasonography in women
  - consideration of prostate-specific antigen in men.

ESR and C-reactive protein

- The ESR measures the rate at which red blood cells aggregate and settle in a test tube. Normal red blood cells repel each other because they carry a net negative charge. Changes in plasma proteins (fibrinogen and globulin) can induce more rapid sedimentation because they are positively charged.
- An elevated ESR is taken as a non-specific sign of, for example, inflammation or malignancy.

- In primary-care populations, the ESR has been found to have a fair discriminating ability with respect to malignancies and inflammatory diseases (sensitivity 53%, specificity 94%).[10] The upper limit for the normal ESR should be set at 12 mm/h for men and 28 mm/h for women, and needs no correction for age.
- Although the ESR is frequently used to rule out disease, it is clear that with such values the ESR is more useful for confirming a diagnosis than excluding the diagnosis of malignancy (*see* SpPin and SnNout in Appendix 1).
- At higher cut-off points the specificity for malignant diseases improves, e.g. for back pain:

	Sensitivity	Specificity
ESR > 20 mm/h	78%	67%
ESR > 50 mm/h	56%	97%

- Thus although at the higher cut-off point there is a greater risk of missing cancers (more false negatives), it is clear that the patients that are identified are much more likely to have disease (SpPin). Considering the relatively low prevalence of malignancies in general practice, a high specificity would be useful.
- C-reactive protein (CRP) is a marker of the acute phase response. Dahler-Eriksen *et al.* concluded that CRP is not a preferred method for diagnosing or monitoring malignant disease.[11]

References

1 Thompson MP and Morris LK (1991) Unexplained weight loss in the ambulatory elderly. *J. Am. Ger. Soc.* **39**: 497–500.

2 Rabinovitz M, Pitlik SD, Leifer M *et al.* (1986) Unintentional weight loss: a retrospective analysis of 154 cases. *Arch. Int. Med.* **146**: 186–7.

3 Marton KI, Sox HC, and Krupp JR (1981) Involuntary weight loss: diagnostic and prognostic significance. *Ann. Int. Med.* **95**: 568–74.

4 Reife CM (1995) Involuntary weight loss. *Med. Clin. North Am.* **79**: 299–313.

5 Deyo RA and Diehl AK (1988) Cancer as a cause of back pain. *J. Gen. Int. Med.* **3**: 230–8.

6 Mazanec DJ (1991) Low back pain syndromes. In: RJ Panzer, ER Black, and PF Griner (eds) *Diagnostic Strategies for Common Medical Problems.* ACP, Philadelphia.

7 Sorensen HT, Mellemkjaer L, Steffensen FH *et al.* (1998) The risk of diagnosis of cancer after primary deep venous thrombosis or pulmonary embolism. *NEJM* **338**: 1169–73.

8   Baron JA, Grindley G, Weiderpass E *et al.* (1998) Venous thromboembolism and cancer. *Lancet* **351**: 1077–80.

9   Buller H and Cate JWT (1998) Primary venous thromboembolism and cancer screening. *NEJM* **338**: 1221–2.

10 Dinant GJ, Knottnerus JA, and Van Wersch JWJ (1991) Discriminating ability of the erythrocyte sedimentation rate: a prospective study in general practice. *Br. J. Gen. Pract.* **41**: 365–70.

11 Dahler-Eriksen BS, Lassen JF, Lund ED *et al.* (1997) C-reactive protein in general practice – how commonly is it used and why? *Scand. J. Prim. Hlth Care* **15**: 35–8.

Appendix 1

Glossary of key terms in clinical epidemiology

- **Incidence:** the incidence refers to the number of new cases of, for example, cancer in a defined population during a specified time period.
- **Prevalence:** the prevalence gives an indication of the numbers of people alive with, for example, cancer in a specified population at a designated time. Hence both the incidence and the longevity of individuals diagnosed with cancer influence the prevalence. Consequently, prevalence measures are most useful for healthcare providers, to assess the public-health impact of a specific disease within a community and to project medical care needs for affected individuals.
- **Predictive value**: the positive predictive value represents the power of an item of clinical information to change the probability that the patient has the disease in question (i.e. the probability that the disease is present if the test is positive). The positive predictive value is synonymous with the term 'posterior probability of the target disorder following a positive test'. The importance for primary care is that the predictive value varies with prevalence – as the prevalence decreases, the proportion of people with the disease decreases and, consequently, the numbers of false positives increase. By analogy, the negative predictive value is the probability that the disease is absent if the test is negative.
- **Posterior probability:** a patient enters the surgery with a prior probability of cancer (i.e. the prevalence of cancer in the population to which they belong, e.g. related to their age, sex, and ethnic origin). Discovering that a patient has, perhaps, a family history of ovarian

cancer alters this risk estimate – the new risk estimate is the posterior probability. This is an example of the application of Bayes's theorem (posterior probability = likelihood ratio × prior odds).

- **Likelihood ratio:** this expresses the odds that a given clinical finding would be expected in a patient with (as opposed to one without) the target disorder. The size of the likelihood ratio gives an indication of the additional 'weight of evidence' that would be provided by the clinical information (i.e. an LR of 14.7 provides more weight than an LR of 2.7, *see* p. 140).
- **Sensitivity:** the proportion of truly diseased persons in the screened population who are identified as diseased by the screening test (i.e. the probability of a positive result in the presence of disease). An associated rule is **SnNout** – if a sign, symptom, or other diagnostic test has sufficiently high sensitivity, a negative result rules out the target disorder (i.e. very few false negatives).
- **Specificity:** the proportion of truly non-diseased persons who are so identified by the screening test (i.e. the probability of a negative result if the disease is absent). An associated rule is **SpPin** – if a sign, symptom, or other diagnostic test has sufficiently high specificity, a positive result rules in the disorder (i.e. very few false positives).
- **Relationships between sensitivity, specificity, and predictive values for the diagnosis of cancer:**

	Cancer present	Cancer absent
Symptom, sign, or diagnostic test result positive	True positive (a)	False positive (b)
Symptom, sign, or diagnostic test result negative	False negative (c)	True negative (d)

Sensitivity = $a/(a + c)$
Specificity = $d/(b + d)$
Positive predictive value = $a/(a + b)$
Negative predictive value = $d/(c + d)$.

- **Screening:** the presumptive identification of unrecognised disease or defects by the application of tests, examinations, or other procedures that can be applied rapidly. Screening programmes need to satisfy a number of criteria (*see* overviews within individual chapters) and to be properly evaluated by randomised controlled trials (RCTs) in order to overcome the potential for bias, in particular lead-time bias.
- **Lead-time bias:** overestimation of survival time, due to the backward shift in the starting point for measuring survival that arises when diseases such as cancer are detected earlier (i.e. the interval between the

diagnosis of a disease by screening and its detection by the development of symptoms).

- **Length-time bias (prevalence–duration bias):** overrepresentation among screen-detected cases of those with a long preclinical phase of disease and thus a more favourable prognosis.

Appendix 2

General sources of information and key contacts in primary-care oncology

Books

Hancock B (1996) *Cancer Care in the Community*. Radcliffe Medical Press, Oxford.

Herold AH and Woodard LJ (1996) *The Medical Clinics of North America: Cancer Screening and Diagnosis*. Vol. 8, No. 1. WB Saunders, Philadelphia.

Hodgkin K (1978) *Towards Earlier Diagnosis in Primary Care*. Churchill Livingstone, London.

Gorroll AH, May LA, and Mulley AG (1995) *Primary Care Medicine. Office Evaluation and Management of the Adult Patient*. Lippincott-Raven, Philadelphia.

Neal AJ and Hoskin PJ (1997) *Clinical Oncology*. Arnold, London.

Panzer RJ, Black ER, and Griner PF (1991) *Diagnostic Strategies for Common Medical Problems*. ACP, Philadelphia.

Sackett DL, Haynes RB, Guyatt GH, and Tugwell P (1991) *Clinical Epidemiology. A Basic Science for Clinical Medicine*. Little, Brown and Co., London.

Schneiderman H and Peixoto AJ (1997) *Bedside Diagnosis*. ACP, Philadelphia.

Organisations

- Agency for Health Care Policy and Research, Executive Office Center, Suite 501, 2101 East Jefferson Street, Rockville, MD 20852, USA

The Agency for Health Care Policy and Research (AHCPR) is a United States government agency established in December 1989 to enhance the quality, appropriateness, and effectiveness of healthcare services and access to these services. The AHCPR guidelines are systematically developed statements to assist practitioner and patient decisions about appropriate healthcare for specific clinical conditions (e.g. No. 18: Smoking cessation).

Accessible from: http://text.nlm.nih.gov/ftrs/dbaccess/capc/
- BACUP, 3 Bath Place, Rivington Street, London, EC2A 3DR, UK
BACUP is a UK charity providing information, emotional support, and counselling to people living with cancer. This website provides information for patients and professionals. The professional section includes a directory of cancer practice guidelines and BACUP's advice to doctors on controversial cancer topics.

Accessible from: http://www.cancerbacup.org.uk/
- Cancer Research Campaign, 10 Cambridge Terrace, London, NW1 4JL, UK
The CRC and its website provide information about publications, appeals, and promotions. There is also patient-oriented information on cancer, including what it is, reducing the risk, and family cancer. Especially valuable are the CRC factsheets, *see* specific references in individual chapters.

Accessible from: http://www.crc.org.uk/
- Christie Cancer Research Centre and the Paterson Institute for Cancer Research, The University of Manchester, Christie Hospital NHS Trust, Wilmslow Road, Withington, Manchester, M20 4BX, UK
Provides information on United Kingdom cancer help groups and associations and a list of cancer research units elsewhere in the United Kingdom.

Accessible from: http:// christie.man.ac.uk
- Department of Health, Richmond House, 79 Whitehall, London, SW1A 2NS, UK
For information on Department of Health Publications (e.g. executive letters and professional letters). Recent publications from the NHS Executive on breast cancer, lung cancer, and colorectal cancer (manuals and research evidence).

Accessible from: http://www.open.gov.uk/doh/dhhome.htm
- Institute of Cancer Research, 17A Onslow Gardens, London, SW7 3AL, UK
The institute and its website offer access to a directory of individual units and research centres and their activities, full text of press releases, and a list of Institute and Hospital publications.

Accessible from:http://www.icr.ac.uk/icrhome.html

- NHS Centre for Reviews and Dissemination, University of York, York, YO1 5DD, UK
  Produces Effective Health Care Bulletins, Effectiveness Matters, and CRD Databases (Database of Abstracts of Reviews of Effectiveness (DARE) and NHS Economic Evaluation Database (NEED)). Recent publications on prostate cancer, lung cancer, breast cancer, and colorectal cancer.
  Accessible from: http://www.york.ac.uk/inst/crd/
- NHS R&D Health Technology Assessment (HTA) Programme, NHS R&D NCCHTA, Bolderwood, University of Southampton, Highfield, Southampton, SO16 7PX, UK
  Recent reviews include prostate cancer and ovarian cancer screening.
  Accessible from: http://www.soton.ac.uk/~hta/index.htm
- Scottish Intercollegiate Guidelines Network (SIGN), Royal College of Physicians of Edinburgh, 9 Queen Street, Edinburgh, EH2 1JQ, UK
  Evidence-based clinical practice guidelines for use by the health service in Scotland. Recent publications on testicular cancer, lung cancer, colorectal cancer, and haematuria.
  Accessible from: http://pc47.cee.hw.ac.uk/sign/graphic.htm

Royal Colleges

The Royal Colleges are often involved in the development of guidelines for specific cancers.
- Royal College of General Practitioners, 14 Princes Gate, Hyde Park, London, SW7 1PU, UK
  http://www.rcgp.org.uk/
- Royal College of Obstetricians and Gynaecologists, St Mary's Hospital, Hathersage Road, Whitworth Park, Manchester, M13 0JH, UK
  http://www.rcog.org.uk/
- Royal College of Physicians of Edinburgh, 9 Queen Street, Edinburgh, EH2 1JQ, UK
  http://www.rcpe.ac.uk
- Royal College of Surgeons of Edinburgh, Nicholson Street, Edinburgh, EH8 9DW, UK
  http://www.rcsed.ac.uk/welcome.htm
- Royal College of Surgeons of England, 35–43 Lincolns Inn Fields, London, WC2A 3PN, UK
  http://www.rcseng.ac.uk

Websites

- CA – a Cancer Journal for Clinicians
  This journal, published bimonthly by Lippincott–Raven for the American Cancer Society, provides primary-care physicians with up-to-date information on all aspects of cancer diagnosis, treatment, and prevention.
  Accessible from: http://www.ca-journal.org/
- CANCERLIT
  Full searching facility for the CANCERLIT bibliographic database, from 1993 to present. The National Cancer Institute's International Cancer Information Center (ICIC) produces the CANCERLIT database by extracting the majority of the cancer-related citations from MEDLINE. This core information is supplemented with additional citations of books, meeting abstracts, theses, and other publications. In addition, the ICIC creates abstracts in CANCERLIT for selected citations that do not contain author abstracts. The database is updated monthly. CANCERLIT citations and abstracts are also searchable from the UK CANCERWEB site.
  Accessible from: http://www.graylab.ac.uk.cancernet/cancerlit/index.html
  http://cnetdb.nci.nih.gov/cancerlit.shtml
- CANCERNET
  Full-text cancer information from the National Cancer Institute (NCI). This includes information statements on treatment, screening, and prevention; patient-orientated information from the NCI's Physician Data Query (PDG) database, and clinical trial data. A full search facility for the CANCERLIT database is also available. A useful feature allows you to use prepared literature searches on more than 90 topics, providing the citations and abstracts for topics added during the previous month. The database is updated monthly.
  Accessible from: http://cancernet.nci.nih.gov/
- Cancer Rates and Risks
  This online publication provides international cancer incidence and mortality rates in a series of charts and graphs. Also included is information on cancer risk factors.
  Accessible from: http://rex.nci.nih.gov/NCI_Pub_Interface/raterisk/index.html
- CANCERWEB
  This cancer resource site has information on many different aspects of cancer, investigation, and treatment. It provides information and resources for patients, healthcare professionals, and scientific

researchers. CANCERWEB includes the CANCERNET and CANCERLIT files.
Accessible from http://www.graylab.ac.uk./cancerweb.html

- European Code Against Cancer
The Code, which gives advice on a healthy lifestyle and early detection of cancer, was originally drawn up by a Committee of Cancer Experts in 1987 and revised in 1994.
Accessible from: http://telescan.nki.nl:80/code/

- *European Journal of Cancer Prevention*
European Journal of Cancer Prevention is the official journal of the European Cancer Prevention Organisation (ECP). It publishes articles on cancer incidence, risk factors, and prevention in the European context.
Accessible from: http://www.chapmanhall.com/cp/default.html

- *Journal of the National Cancer Institute Online*
This service provides abstracts for major articles on cancer.
Accessible from: http://cancernet.nci.nih.gov/jnci/jnci_issues.html

- Oncolink
A multimedia online cancer information resource provided by the University of Pennsylvania. Oncolink is aimed at a wide audience, including healthcare professionals and patients. The service is a mixture of original information and links to information at other sites (especially the National Cancer Institute) and allows browsing (by disease or medical speciality) and keyword searching.
Accessible from: http://cancer.med.upenn.edu/

- Oncoweb
Oncoweb is a free, online educational resource and information service for professionals working in the oncology field. This resource is provided by the European School of Oncology, and Greenwich Medical Online. The European Association for Cancer Research home page can be found on this site, as well as the searchable and browsable START database of oncology treatment. Other information provided includes conference details, case studies, and links with related cancer sites. The content of the pages are reviewed by the OncoWeb Editorial Board, comprised of oncology specialists.
Accessible from: http://www.oncoweb.com/

Major medical journals on the web

- *BMJ*: http://www.bmj.com/
- *Journal of the American Medical Association* (JAMA): http://www.ama-assn.org.sci-pubs/journals/most/recent/issues/jama/toc.htm

- The *Lancet* Interactive: http://www.thelancet.com/
- *New England Journal of Medicine*: http://www.nejm.org/

Appendix 3

MEDLINE searches for diagnostic studies on ESR, 1985–94

MeSH terms	Number of citations
#1 BLOOD-SEDIMENTATION/all subheadings	
#2 HEMORHEOLOGY/all s.	
#3 explode ACUTE-PHASE-PROTEINS/diagnostic use	
#4 (#1 or #2 or #3) and ((TG=human or TG=male or TG=female))	
#5 explode DIAGNOSIS/all s.	
#6 explode DIAGNOSIS/diagnosis	
#7 DIAGNOSIS-DIFFERENTIAL/all s.	
#8 explode SENSITIVITY-AND-SPECIFICITY	
#9 REFERENCE-VALUES/all s.	
#10 FALSE-NEGATIVE-REACTIONS/all s.	
#11 FALSE-POSITIVE-REACTIONS/all s.	
#12 explode MASS-SCREENING/all s.	
#13 #5 or #8 or #9 or #10 or #11 or #12 (extended version)	
#14 #6 or #7 or #8 or #9 or #10 or #11 or #12 (short version)	
#15 #4 and #13 (extended version)	1387
#16 #4 and #14 (short version)	201
#17 FAMILY-PRACTICE/all s.	
#18 PHYSICIANS-FAMILY/all s.	

#19   explode PRIMARY-HEALTH-CARE/all s.
#20   #16 and (#17 or #18 or #19)   8

Freetext terms:
#21   (sedimentation near blood) or (sedimentation near erythrocyte).
#22   #21 and (TG=human or TG=male or TG=female)
#23   diagnos*
#24   sensitivity or specificity
#25   predictive value*
#26   reference value*
#27   ROC*
#28   likelihood ratio*
#29   monitoring
#30   #23 or #24 or #25 or #26 or #27 or #28 or #29
#31   #22 and #30
#32   #15 or #31 (combined search)
#33   ((family practi*) or (family physician*))
#34   ((general practi* or (primary health care))
#35   #31 and (#33 or #34)
#36   #20 or #35

* = $ = truncation.
DIAGNOSIS-DIFFERENTIAL is covered by explode DIAGNOSIS.
PREDICTIVE-VALUE-OF-TESTS   and   ROC-CURVE   are   covered   by
explode SENSITIVITY-AND-SPECIFICITY.

Reference

Weijden T, Ijzermans CJ, Dinant GJ *et al.* (1997) Identifying relevant diagnostic studies in *Medline*. The diagnostic value of the erythrocyte sedimentation rate (ESR) and dipstick as an example. *Fam. Pract.* **14**: 204–8.

Index

α-fetoprotein (AFP) 82
β-human chorionic gonadotrophin (β-HCG) 82

abdominal symptoms
  colorectal cancer 30, 31, 32–3
  upper gastrointestinal cancers 104–5
actinic keratoses 128, 129, 130
acute lymphoblastic leukaemia (ALL)
  epidemiology 107–8
  incidence 7
  investigations in primary care 111
  pathology and prognosis 108
  symptoms and signs in primary care 110
  treatment 109
acute myeloid leukaemia (AML)
  epidemiology 107–8
  investigations in primary care 111
  pathology and prognosis 108
  risk factors 108
  symptoms and signs in primary care 110
  treatment 109
adenocarcinoma 10
adenomatosis polyposis coli (APC) 10, 24
Aflatoxin 11
age factors 5
  bladder cancer 71

breast cancer 49, 50
cervical cancer 95
colorectal cancer 23, 30–1, 32
genetic predisposition to cancer 9
head and neck cancer 119
incidence 6–7
leukaemia 107–8
lung cancer 39
lymphoma 112
melanoma 131
multiple myeloma 116
ovarian cancer 85
prostate cancer 63, 68
testicular cancer 79
upper gastrointestinal cancers 101
Agency for Health Care Policy and Research 149–50
airflow obstruction 46
American College of Obstetricians and Gynecologists 93
anaemia
  colorectal cancer 31–2
  kidney 75, 76
  multiple myeloma 118
androgen-deprivation therapy 65
ankylosing spondylitis 108
Ann Arbor staging
  Hodgkin's disease 113
  non-Hodgkin's lymphoma 114
anovulation 85